ELKE GERAERTS

THE MENTAL RESET

How hybrid work and life
strengthen your resilience

Lannoo

Contents

CHAPTER 3
BUILD BACK BETTER
How to take control of your own life

CHAPTER 4

THE BRAIN IS KEY IN THE NEW WAY OF WORKING

Why hybrid work is here to stay

CHAPTER 5

THE MOST HYBRID EMPLOYER OF THE YEAR

A new era requires new leaders

CHAPTER 6
THE FUTURE IS ALREADY HERE
Why brain-friendly policies are also for the young

INTRODUCTION

MY BIG RESET

28 March 2020. It was a moment that sent shivers down my spine. In amongst the doom-laden news about Covid, a video clip caught my attention. Opera singer Sarah Defrise Nirenburg and her pianist partner gave a concert on the patio outside their home in Brussels. As arias by Gershwin and Puccini filled the air, neighbours emerged one by one. They leaned out of the windows of anonymous blocks of flats or stood close together in their household bubble on tiny balconies. Some daredevils even climbed the walls of their urban gardens to get a better glimpse of the opera singer. Each song was greeted with loud applause, with the decibels increasing every time, so it seemed. I watched the video again and again, moved by how the neighbours reached out to one another, each on their own island and yet still with that connection. I saw hope, beauty and emotion. I drew strength from the way that people in full lockdown never gave up. Despite the crisis we were in, there was still so much to be happy about.

In the days that followed, I recharged my batteries with similar video clips. I was touched by how the people of Italy, at that point the worst affected country in the world, sang from their balconies to give one another courage. The author Ilja Leonard Pfeijffer, who lives in Genoa, put it neatly in his Covid diary: "It was an unexpected sign of life and resilience. It turned out there were fellow sufferers behind all those closed windows. The streets had been deserted for days, but the people were still there. For the five minutes that the concert lasted, they kept up their courage and comforted one another by showing they were still alive."

I also became addicted to the live Instagram videos of the Italian Michelin-star chef Massimo Bottura, who had to temporarily close his restaurant in Modena because of the coronavirus. Instead, he took to showing his 1.2 million followers what was cooking in his pots and pans every evening. In his Kitchen Quarantine clips, we saw his human side as well as his passion for his profession. There he was, preparing ordinary everyday dishes for his family. The top chef did not hide the fact that his youngest son Charlie has a mental disability either — it doesn't get more authentic than that. It was also surprisingly comforting to see Massimo preparing his fresh pasta with tomato sauce after a hard day at work.

His videos inspired me to start my own new habit. We were all finding it really difficult that my parents were unable to see their grandchildren during the lockdown. Normally they see one another every week. Also, I'm their only daughter. So I decided to instigate a brief FaceTime session with them around the children's bedtime. I would normally find daily video calls rather boring but now it soon became a good way to feel some kind of connection. Even if the girls were sometimes dropping off to sleep — Florence and Feline were only five and six — and we didn't always say much, it was still a special moment. I experienced at first hand every day that even in a crisis, you can still begin something new. It was the start of my mental reset.

It promised to be a major reset. The Covid crisis wiped out the schedule for my company, Better Minds at Work, in one fell swoop. While the costs continued unabated — I refused to furlough my staff — I found myself as the CEO dealing with entrepreneurial risks such as I had never experienced in my previous career in academia. My private life was even more turbulent. My marriage fell apart just before the first lockdown. In the first few months of the pandemic, my ex and I were still living in the same house. The restrictions were literally preventing me from leaving. But I felt rejuvenated by the idea that I would soon be making a new start.

However, I did not realize how difficult the months ahead would be. Although I know a lot of people who have gone through a divorce, it felt as if no one had ever told me how hard that is when children are involved. There is so much sadness and distress. After I had moved out, it felt inconceivably unnatural having to drop the girls off at their father's house every week. I had not anticipated the pain of no longer being a family. The weekends without the girls felt very empty, a feeling that was exacerbated by the Covid measures.

After a few weekends of inactivity and wallowing in misery, I decided this had to stop. By giving in to the pain, I was sinking deeper and deeper in a negative spiral. I knew this wasn't going to put an end to my misery or help me process things, so I looked for activities that would give me energy. Instead of spending my Saturday mornings on Netflix, I started the day with 15 minutes of yoga. Instead of chomping down a fatty snack, I jumped on my racing bike. And when I didn't have enough stamina to give it my all on my bike, I went for a walk in the fresh air. I often took my first book, *Better Minds*, with me. Everything I had once written about resilience I now put into practice. For example, I tried to pause and examine my thoughts. What was I thinking about? How rational were those thoughts? What kind of a vicious circle had I got into?

Slowly but surely, I turned my crisis into a source of strength. Now, in November 2021, not only does Better Minds at Work have a full schedule again but I have a new book. I have become more of a hands-on mother for my children and in the relational sphere I have found happiness again with Bert. Thanks to my mental reset and the years I had invested in my mental capital, I was able to rapidly rebuild my life... and improve it. "Build Back Better", as the US president Joe Biden would say.

In this book, I want to show how everyone, from individuals to companies and from teenagers to politicians, can use a crisis as a catalyst for positive change. Nor does it stop there. My ambition is for *Mental Reset* to become a model for growth, quite apart from the Covid pandemic or any other crisis. I want this book not just to inform you but also to inspire you to reset your own life. Reset in the sense of building back better. I call it bouncing forward rather than bouncing back. The key is investing in your mental capital, preferably proactively. And you do that by concentrating on resilience.

In the first two chapters, I focus on the challenges we are facing and how we can convert them into opportunities. Then I call on our governments to do more to facilitate future changes in ways that take into account how our brains work. The real work begins in the third chapter, where I give mental levers for a successful reset.

In the next two chapters, I examine in more depth what work will look like in the future and how we can make brain-aware choices. Few areas of our lives were affected so dramatically by the pandemic as work. Many people experienced at first hand how exhausting working from home can be. But there is huge potential in hybrid working — switching flexibly between home and the office and preferably with a whole range of individual options for employees. Hybrid working is the future, but that will require a major mindset shift for a lot of companies. A new era also needs new leaders. In Chapter 5, I consider what that new leadership should look like and explore how we can really get the best out of hybrid companies and other organizations.

I have devoted my final chapter to the young, a group that was hit by this crisis just when they were in an important stage of their development. Too often they have been called 'a lost generation', whereas I have high hopes that they will become a particularly empathic, resilient generation. That won't just happen automatically of course, which is why I explicitly address people working in education and policy in this chapter. After all, the post-Covid era is not just a chance for individual employees and companies to make a mental reset, but also the perfect opportunity for our education system to make brain-aware choices.

'Brain-aware' is a term you will encounter repeatedly throughout this book. I never cease to be surprised at the fact that although we have known for years what we should do to make choices for our brains that give us long-term happiness and success, we still fail to put this into practice. Yet in the strange eighteen months we have just been through, I also saw how we suddenly adopted a whole new way of living and working. So that reset *is* possible.

That is the message I want to get across with this book. Things will never be the same again — and thank goodness for that! This new era offers us more possibilities than ever before to take a different, hybrid approach to our lives and our work. Hopefully my book will inspire you to embrace that hybrid life and make your own distinctive version.

CHAPTER 1

MAKE IT COUNT

WHY THE GOOD OLD DAYS WEREN'T NECESSARILY THAT GREAT

"Iceland now feels like the corona crisis never happened," was a CNN headline in June 2020. In May 2021, I read on Vox that "Bosses are acting like the pandemic never happened" and in January 2021 Belgian newspaper *De Morgen's* China correspondent Leen Vervaeke wrote an article with the title "As if nothing happened. That is Wuhan today." Of course, I too am pleased I can go out for a meal with my friends again and the children can restart their swimming lessons, but I find media headlines like this rather depressing nevertheless. We seem to have forgotten that the pre-Covid world had its problems too. Many people see COVID-19 as the main reason for the brain crisis that is spreading and worsening. People feel drained and exhausted, there is a seemingly unstoppable epidemic of burnout and depression, and loneliness is affecting young and old. But we forget that in terms of our mental health, red lights were already flashing before COVID-19. Some people actually found life and work easier during the coronavirus crisis because it briefly brought the dreaded rat race to a stop.

Our brains have been under pressure for a long time

The World Health Organization (WHO) published the following dizzying figures. Nearly one billion people have a psychiatric disorder and everyone runs a risk of it, regardless of where they are in the world. Depression is a key cause of invalidity around the world and is a major factor in the global sickness burden. An estimated 5 per cent of the adult population worldwide suffer from depression. One in seven youngsters aged 10 to 19 has a mental disorder. Half of these disorders start around the age of 14 but most remain undetected and untreated. Suicides account for one in a hundred deaths. Suicide is the fourth biggest cause of death for young people aged between 15 and 29.

The loss of productivity due to depression and anxiety costs the global economy an estimated one trillion dollars. Compare that with the fact that countries spend only 2 per cent of their national healthcare budgets on mental health.

Despite all these dizzying figures, there has been little change in the past few years. Hopefully the pandemic will finally spark off a turnaround, but at present it has primarily led to long waiting lists for psychologists and a shortage of beds for long-term mental health treatment. In my own circle, I know of a young person who was struggling with suicidal thoughts and had to wait for a year. Another person had addiction issues and also had to wait a year to get help. If you don't have the money to pay for an expensive psychiatrist in private health, you have nowhere to go. There is crisis help, but it often doesn't amount to much more than occupational therapy. Two weeks later, you're sent home.

It is shocking to see how much money and attention there is for our physical health and how little for our mental health. This pressure our brains are under urgently needs to be tackled, but that in itself is not enough. Whenever you have such pressure, you also need the courage to focus on prevention.

Fanning the flames

In short, the pandemic was not the main culprit behind the mental health crisis; the situation was already perilous. But COVID-19 — and especially how we dealt with the pandemic — did fan the flames. Vigorously. A year and a half of social isolation, stress, uncertainty and the (perfectly legitimate) fear of catching the disease: the coronavirus crisis tested our resilience to the utmost. There were no vaccines or other solutions available at first, and for a long time we had no idea when or how we would ever be able to resume our normal lives. On top of that, the crisis was unexpected and no one was properly prepared.

Given all this, it is hardly surprising that many people became caught in a vicious circle of negativity. Especially when you think that our primeval brain — that part of our brain that is geared to survival and is hypersensitive to danger — happens to like wallowing in negative news.

BWAH DE VIVRE

"I don't recognize myself. I'm normally quite a positive type but now I can't stop worrying." Does that sound like you? Or have you found the coronavirus crisis took a toll on your mental health in other ways? You will be pleased to hear that in many cases the problem is temporary, without any long-term effect on your mental wellbeing. "After most potentially traumatic experiences, the vast majority of people will only see a temporary, limited impact on their mental health," clinical psychology professor Patrick Luyten assures us in a newspaper article. Minimal-impact resilience is the norm, he says.

Nearly everyone experienced minor symptoms. The *New York Times* called "languishing" the dominant emotion in 2021. Languishing means feeling 'blah'. *Bwah de vivre*, as a caller on a Brussels radio programme so fittingly called it. In the face of a life that seemed to have lost its élan, we became flat and apathetic. While before Covid we sometimes complained about an excess of stimuli, now we suffered from a lack of novelty. It was the same old, same old. Each caught in our individual bubble, we were all stripped of our sparkle.

One effect of this life devoid of stimuli is deterioration in our cognitive powers. To give an example, in June 2021 I saw a photo on Instagram of a friend who was about to set off for an exotic island. Normally I'm the type who loves to travel but now I caught myself thinking: what a hassle, definitely not for me. It seemed cognitively demanding to have to apply for the right documents and have my trip depend on the results of a PCR test. And yet in 2018 I didn't find it a problem to go through the visa application process for Saint Petersburg, which was an awful lot more hassle than a simple PCR test. But now arranging that test for my family seemed an almost impossible task.

You can compare the cognitive deterioration with the symptoms of bore-out or when children are locked away in a room and deprived of stimulation for months on end. In the past year "everyone we know has gone a little bit Kaspar Hauser", wrote columnist Eleanor Margolis in *The Guardian*, referring to the German boy who turned up after spending sixteen years in solitary confinement in the early nineteenth century.

Fortunately, our brains are quite flexible and resilient. You can recover from the cognitive deterioration by gradually adjusting to normal life again, picking up the threads little by little so that your mental pathways can rearrange themselves. The phrase "little by little" is very important. Some people may have discovered first hand that it is not a good idea to throw yourself in the deep end, when their first day back at the office also included their first post-pandemic train journey and their first visit to a cafe for drinks with co-workers.

All those stimuli can make you feel like your head is about to explode. That is perfectly normal, says psychologist and happiness expert Josje Smeets. "Our brains have adapted to the long lockdown with very few stimuli. When you are then suddenly exposed to repeated extreme stimulation, for example because you are partying a lot, your brain will go into stress mode." That does not mean we should not take this issue seriously. "In the longer term, this can damage your mental health and may even lead to burnout."

Psychiatrist Dirk De Wachter also recommends taking time to readjust. "I hope I don't sound like an old fogey but we need to pace ourselves. So we should be cautious rather than plunging back into life with loads of activities after Covid. Don't get obsessed with the idea 'I have to do it now'. Slowly build up the partying and nightlife; plan pauses in your diary. Not because I say so but because your mind needs it."

The good news is that the habits that we want to pick up again may have been on hold for a while but they have not disappeared from our memory for good. Just as you don't forget how to ski if you miss a year, so the habits of shaking hands, socializing at a family do or going crazy at a rock concert haven't withered away in our brains. While we soon got used to not giving people a hug when we met them, and even found it strange to see characters hugging in films during lockdown, we will equally quickly find it perfectly normal once it is allowed again. The hugging habit is still wired into our brains and can be reactivated relatively rapidly.

THE DISILLUSION OF FREEDOM

"At first I couldn't understand why my girlfriend found the pandemic so much harder going than I did," a colleague said to me. "But then I realized that as an extrovert she really missed the social contacts whereas I am an introvert and was quite happy to spend more time on my own, in fact. Now our social lives have resumed, our diaries are full once again with dinners with friends. I never used to have a problem with that but now I sometimes catch myself balking at those evenings."

For some people, rather than harming their mental health, Covid brought relief. They enjoyed the peace and quiet, exercised more, ate more healthily and felt mentally stronger. Having to face the busy world again is a challenge for introverts or people with autism. Highly sensitive people may also experience a setback at this stage. What if their employer expects them to return to the office three days a week, proposing two days working from home as a privilege? What if they no longer feel able to cope with the hustle and bustle at the office and the stress of the commute?

During the pandemic, many people discovered there were things they would rather no longer do in future. When the amusement parks opened again in the spring of 2021, I stood in a line of hundreds of people queuing to get into Walibi near Brussels. "Great! Rollercoasters and quality time with my daughters," I'd thought that morning. We three had been looking forward to this day out for a long time, but as we stood in the queue I felt more and more despondent by the minute. How was that possible? When I had looked forward to the trip for so long?

It was hugely disillusioning — until I realized I wouldn't have been jumping for joy in the queue before Covid either. I realized that as an introvert I no longer felt up to this at all. I had found life a lot more fun in my little cocoon for the past eighteen months than I ever did on a rollercoaster full of people shrieking.

I am sure I'm not the only person who was longing for the return to normal like a delicious ice cream only to discover to their disappointment that it didn't taste as good as expected. We are who we are. And that is fine: there is no need for all of us to be real extroverts. But we do need to take responsibility for our own happiness. A proactive person will not have spent the entire coronavirus crisis complaining that they missed the contact with their co-workers. No, they will have arranged to go on walks together or have had long conversations by phone.

I have been here before. In 2006, I moved to the US for a job at Harvard University. I saw America as the promised land. "All the *éminences grises* in psychology will be on my corridor," I said to myself in anticipation. I told everyone, "I won't be coming back". I sold my house and gave all the contents to my boyfriend at the time. But when I looked in the mirror in Boston, I soon realized that I was still the same person. Even in this 'promised land', it would be up to me, with all my strengths and weaknesses, to make something of it. People often forget that aspect. No new country or crisis exit strategy is going to solve all your problems

LOCKDOWN TRAUMAS

In addition to the excess stimulation and disillusionment of the post-Covid period, there are other mental health effects of the coronavirus crisis that are still to come. Many people who experience trauma only display symptoms after six months or more. A 'post-traumatic stress disorder with delayed onset' is the term we use in psychology. We can expect that wave soon.

The coronavirus crisis as trauma. Some people, especially the elderly, laugh that off. The war was a real trauma, they say. But the pandemic and the Second World War have quite a lot of similarities. In both cases, the crisis was unexpected and was accompanied by a great deal of uncertainty and fear. No one knew how long it would continue. Trauma expert Berthold Gersons agrees that the coronavirus pandemic is comparable to a disaster: "It hit us all of a sudden, it was life-threatening, there were victims and it led to a feeling of insecurity, chaos and dependence on others to be able to survive." A disaster with one very strange feature, moreover: "There is very little expression of grief. People are restraining themselves." According to Gersons, that is because it was not clear when the danger had receded. "In nearly all disasters, there comes a point when people know they are safe again. You can leave the spot and then it's over. You know that those are the victims and you are not one of them. But here no one knows whether they will survive it in the end," he said in an interview with Dutch newspaper *De Volkskrant*.

A post-traumatic stress disorder (PTSD) can manifest itself in various ways. A common symptom is intrusive thoughts. By that I mean that from time to time you unexpectedly fall prey to negative memories of the traumatic event. That happens to me on occasion now when I'm at the office. I suddenly think back to the webinars I gave to an empty office during the first lockdown. All the negative feelings from that period come rushing back: the uncertainty about the financial position of Better Minds at Work, the problems on the home front. "It's all OK, it is in the past," I whisper to reassure myself. Nightmares with flashbacks are another possible symptom, along with cognitive problems such as difficulty concentrating. PTSD can also affect your sleep or your mood. However, people find the repetitive, difficult-to-control thoughts most troublesome.

The best method for processing trauma is confrontation. Of course, that is difficult if the trauma concerns an event in the past. You can put people with a fear of flying on a plane to help them overcome their fear but we can't really put people with Covid PTSD back in lockdown. However, the confrontation can also take the form of a thought exercise. For example, a trauma therapist will often ask a patient with PTSD questions to take them back to the situation and their feelings at the time, then make them aware of the silver linings as a way of weakening the trauma.

Who are particularly susceptible to a depression or PTSD as a result of the pandemic? Who are the people who say that the coronavirus crisis did not have a single positive effect on their lives? Your genetic disposition is always a factor — some people's DNA makes them less resilient to traumatic experiences than others. Upbringing plays a role too. If your parents always applied a pessimistic explanatory style throughout your childhood, you may well adopt the same style. On the other hand, this may have irritated you so much that you expressly try to counter their behaviour by doing the exact opposite.

VALET PARKING

Anyone who has ever listened to one of my talks or read any of my previous books will know that I am a fervent advocate of living your life in the driver's seat. Taking ownership of your life is so important for your mental resilience. But I sometimes wonder whether we have forgotten how to do this due to Covid. While there was criticism of the coronavirus measures and illegal lockdown parties regularly made the headlines, the overwhelming majority of the population here in Belgium were very obedient. We stayed indoors after ten at night, made sure we didn't have more than one guest in our homes and continued disinfecting our shopping trolleys long after it was proven that the virus mainly infected people through airborne contact. At the start of the crisis, even the press — which can normally be relied upon to criticize anything and everything — acted as if they were the spokespeople for the scientists and the government. This acquiescence surprised me. I had expected the restaurants to spontaneously open again as an act of civil disobedience, but that didn't happen.

Don't get me wrong: of course I'm not saying the measures should have been ignored. But I do think we should investigate why it is that individuals demonstrated so little ownership because this is confirmation of a trend I have noticed for some time. We are so eager to give someone else the blame, but we also effortlessly hand over control of our lives as if the government is a valet who will park our car safely for us while we check into our comfort zone. Many people behaved like wronged underdogs, complaining that life is not fair. Agreed, that is often the case. But if you act like an underdog, you will never achieve anything. In fact, it will only make you less happy. Ownership and autonomy are important prerequisites for mental wellbeing.

See the clip about the driver's seat
on the Mental Reset video channel.

Resilience is the key

Do we really want to go back to the old normal? Or would we prefer to finally find a solution to our old problems in this new, post-Covid world. My sincere wish is that the coronavirus does have a lasting impact. I don't want us to simply return to how things were; I want us to draw lessons from the crisis and work on the future based on these new insights. Otherwise that period really will have been lost time. I hope that as individuals and as society as a whole we don't go back to our everyday lives on autopilot, but instead proactively deal with this next stage and personally take ownership.

How can we do that? By working on our resilience. The *Herald of Free Enterprise* ferry disaster taught us that post-traumatic stress is not the only possible outcome, as some of the survivors were actually found to have experienced post-traumatic growth.

The deciding factor was resilience. Resilience determines how we deal with setbacks and consequently how susceptible we are to stress and burnout. In my doctoral research at Maastricht University, I investigated resilience among the victims of child abuse and among war veterans. These were all people who had suffered serious blows in life but who had also often demonstrated huge resilience. The good news is that such resilience isn't just something you are born with: you can also train your mental resilience. This insight was one of the founding ideas of my book *Better Minds.*

That's right — you yourself can decide to become mentally resilient and actively control your life rather than being swept up in the misery and blaming others. What does this get you? You will be able to get through a long period of setbacks without losing your balance, recover relatively quickly and perhaps flourish more than ever as a result.

That is precisely why I see this crisis as a major opportunity. I started Better Minds at Work because I wanted to show people that they have more resilience than they think. That notion often met with a lot of resistance; people didn't believe me. We often assume we are unable to cope with trials and tribulations. Yet now we have demonstrated *en masse* that we are all resilient to some degree. Even if the crisis had continued for another year, most of us would have kept going. For me too, resilience has become more tangible in the past year. Previously, I had often studied the phenomenon as a theoretical concept, but during the coronavirus crisis I could see and feel it everywhere. I constantly saw confirmation of my gut feeling.

As you saw, my own resilience was sorely tested in the early days of the pandemic. But once I started to consistently apply the levers I describe in my book *Better Minds*, I regained control of the situation.

LEVER 1

Self-awareness

In the first place, I tried to become aware of my thoughts. For example, one night I lay awake worrying how I should tell everyone the news if the difficult financial situation continued much longer and I had to make some of my staff redundant. I was able to distance myself from my thoughts by asking myself the question. "What are you thinking?" I realized this was irrational. Why would the crisis continue so much longer? Even if that was the case, why would it mean that companies no longer wanted to make use of our expertise? By taking a sheet of paper and listing my fears on the left and the facts on the right, I could see at a glance that my thoughts had got out of hand. I was catastrophizing: one of the thought patterns — along with polarized thinking and overgeneralization, for instance — that we get caught up in when we are anxious. And sure enough, I was proved wrong. From November, the continuing crisis prompted an increase in demand for our services and by January we were even having to turn clients away. The worries I had in March 2020 turned out to be groundless. Fortunately I was able to put a stop to these worries in good time by recognizing and explicitly identifying this thought pattern.

I practised that same meta-awareness when scheduling my work. For example, I don't like doing sessions on autopilot. I try to avoid this wherever possible because mindlessly repeating a lesson is not what it's about for me. Yet perhaps 200 sessions of the 'Better Minds' webinar were planned for the past year. As if I was a robot you could switch on and off. When I realized dozens of online sessions were scheduled in my diary, I proactively approached the managers who had booked me and asked them to link to me in LinkedIn and send me feedback and questions. That often meant extra work that I wasn't obliged to do and was free of charge for the client. But that connection is one aspect that motivates me. If I get feedback after a talk or hear what an impact the session had on the client, this energizes me and helps me repeat the talk time and time again. It leaves me glowing, with my batteries fully recharged. An online session where you neither hear nor see another soul, on the other hand, saps my energy levels.

SELF-AWARENESS

We spend almost half our time – about 47 per cent of the day – with our thoughts not on what we are doing. Our mind is elsewhere. That is not necessarily a bad thing. Take Archimedes with his eureka moment in his bath. To be creative, we need times when our thoughts roam freely. But unfortunately it is also true that the less control we have over our thoughts, the worse we feel. After all, our thoughts have a tendency to sink down a negative rabbit hole. Thinking about thinking is one of the most efficient techniques for increasing our self-awareness. If you actively ask yourself, "What am I thinking about?" from time to time, you will become more aware of your thought patterns. It will let you put a stop to negative thoughts or turn them into positive ones.

See the clip about self-awareness
on the Mental Reset video channel.

LEVER 2

Focus

In addition to practising self-awareness, I also made sure to keep my focus. One way I did this was in setting clear priorities. For example, I soon realized that I wanted to spend more time with my children. Before the pandemic, I was on the go throughout the working week. I would often leave early in the morning and only get back home after the children had gone to bed. I saw the school run as a waste of time: I had Justine, our nanny, for that. But the coronavirus control measures meant I suddenly had to do that myself. What is more, Justine broke her foot around the same time. One morning, we passed the place where it happened. My younger daughter asked me when Justine would be returning. I told her that she wouldn't. "Of course, that's right," she said. "You're looking after us now and that's much nicer."

How could I deprive them of that again? By telling them I have to give a talk at the other end of the country? And to be honest, I wouldn't want to miss the school run anymore. These days it feels like quality time rather than a chore. So I try to keep that time free now. For example, a company asked me whether I could come to their studio in Amsterdam to give an online talk for 500 teachers. I have excellent Wi-Fi at home so I told them, "Find a solution". In the past, I would have been much more inclined to accommodate them, but now I don't see the added value of those extra hours travelling if I can also give the talk online from my office at home and thereby spend more time with my children. Moreover, I don't find it so difficult to set limits because I know what my priorities are.

FOCUS

People who are focused are more alert, worry less and experience less stress. However, focus has become like gold dust in a world where the apps on our smartphones are constantly competing for our attention. In the past decade, our attention span has plummeted because of this.

Setting priorities is one of the most powerful ways to sharpen our focus. Setting long-term objectives is the only way to avoid being carried away by the latest hype. That and developing a strategy to control the tsunami of information.

See the clip about focus
on the Mental Reset video channel.

LEVER 3

Self-control and willpower

In addition to self-awareness and focus, I also bolstered my self-control and willpower. Instead of just lounging around during the lockdown, I decided to use this unexpected free time to write a book as a way of doing something that would feel satisfying and reap benefits in the longer term. After all, now I had the space to do that.

Rather than going into pause mode and wallowing in the status quo of the crisis, I tried to work proactively on myself in those areas of my life where this was possible. Unfortunately, many people did not do this. They put their lives on hold and waited for the pandemic to end, whereas they should have done the exact opposite to strengthen their resilience. As a result, life lost its sparkle for them. Some ended up in a languishing state, a sensation suspended somewhere between depression and happiness. Companies also ended up in a similar state. Because many companies did not really plan ahead, they were left fighting a losing battle on employee welfare from November 2020. They realized far too late that they would have to maintain the new regime for much longer, that the crisis was a marathon rather than a sprint, and that they would not reach the finish unless they changed tack. After all, willpower is not inexhaustible. That was clear among the general public by Christmas 2020. Everyone had their own interpretation of the measures, but very few families stuck strictly to the rules. They thought they were allowed to make an exception… as long as their neighbours didn't follow suit. For me, that was a sign of things to come. Their willpower was stretched to the limit.

I know that willpower is not inexhaustible so I made sure to arrange my life so that I would be able to keep up this situation for a long time. If you have to suppress your desires too often, you run a real risk of succumbing to them in the end. There were no prospects of improvement in the world outside, so I turned my attention to my own cocoon. Rather than focusing on all the things that were not allowed, I looked at the situation from a different perspective. What *was* still allowed? That was how I decided to invite someone every weekend to go for a walk with me. That might seem rather banal, but it meant I always had something to look forward to. It motivated me and stopped me from being tempted to break the rules.

SELF-CONTROL

What do all truly successful people have in common? They don't give up when they have a setback, and they tend to constantly look for new challenges. Because they are aware of the impact their actions have in the long term, they have no problem withstanding the temptations of everyday life.

Self-control is something you preferably learn as a child, but adults can also increase their willpower by looking for activities that they find intrinsically motivating and address their 'why' question. But no one has inexhaustible willpower. That is why you need to build in sufficient pauses to recharge your batteries.

See the clip about self-control
on the Mental Reset video channel.

LEVER 4
Optimism

That brings me to the final lever for resilience: optimism. How you see a situation determines how it makes you feel. I was able to get through the crisis year well by looking at what I could still do and by setting things in motion.

I was sorry to see some people develop a real obsession with the dreaded virus. Rather than following every twist and turn in its progress on the news or searching for all the information about COVID-19, I simply kept to the rules as best I could. I deliberately concentrated on activities and friends that cheered me up rather than listening to the latest news update full of doom and gloom. Before I went to sleep, I would run through all the positive events and hopeful stories of that day. I made sure my list was long enough: you need four positive things to outweigh one negative thing. Does that mean I waltzed through 2020 buoyed by naivety and false positivism? No, not at all. I too felt despondent at times and wondered whether it would ever be over. If I was struggling, I made sure people could see that. However, I also managed to give my feelings a more positive slant simply through my thought patterns and the activities I chose.

OPTIMISM

Don't confuse optimism with a naive belief that things will end well. It is not the same, and that belief can even be dangerous. Unlike pessimists, optimists have a positive explanatory style. If something goes wrong, you will never hear them say things always go wrong. They will never sigh and ask why this always has to happen to them. Instead, they will see it as a challenge and respond accordingly. Optimists also differ from pessimists in how they react to stress. Optimists confront their problems whereas pessimists stick their heads in the sand.

You can foster an optimistic attitude by actively seeking out things and people that make you feel good. Relationships, meaningfulness and creativity are also key factors in determining our happiness.

See the clip about optimism
on the Mental Reset video channel.

In short, I kept my resilience levers intact during the coronavirus crisis, but a new dimension was added: I saw how important it is to be proactive, not to go into pause mode during a crisis but to speed up the transformation instead. And while it made me realize more than ever that you need to take responsibility for how you emerge from a crisis, that is of course not the whole story. Our resilience is also partly determined by our genes, our upbringing and everything we have been through. There is no panacea that works for everyone, but an open mindset is a good start. Our schools, companies and politicians also have a major role to play. I will consider this in greater depth later in the book.

The Great Return

"I expect everyone to be back in the office on Monday, as we will be restarting then." A friend told me that she and her co-workers felt so put off by this e-mail from her manager that they asked him to postpone the Great Return. "Restarting": did that mean her manager wanted to go back to the old ways, that he didn't want to make *any* substantial changes?

Her boyfriend's company had taken a much better approach. In keeping with the UEFA Euro 2020 spirit, all the employees at DPG Media were given a personalized football shirt for their 'reboarding'. This made the return to the office something festive, a new start and an opportunity to wipe the slate clean and reconfigure working life. Not a 'restart' but a genuine reset.

In my personal life too, resets — in other words, starting afresh with a clean sheet — are my go-to growth model. I've done this a couple of times already. For ten years, my academic career was my reference point in my life. I lived and breathed my research and I collaborated with the leading figures in my discipline. But there came a point when I noticed that my enthusiasm was waning. It was always the same cycle of lecturing, publishing articles and presenting papers at conferences. I did a lot of scientific research but often without any obvious impact, as if I was pouring energy into a container that then closed. It seemed as if all I was doing was building an impressive CV. Eventually I decided I would quit and set up my own company. There are no entrepreneurs in my family and no one seemed to understand why I was doing this. I had a generous employment contract guaranteeing me a job until I retired and I was on course to become a professor. Why in Heaven's name make this change? My father said I was crazy to give up such a fantastic career. My colleagues were surprised too. Why not get a change of scene by moving to another university? Surely you don't want to waste all those years of study and research? But I knew that if I did continue, I would end up having a bore-out. My work no longer addressed my personal 'why' — helping people and making an impact. So I went from being a government employee at the university in Rotterdam to running my own business in Antwerp, a city where I knew no one. It was a huge step that needed a lot of courage to take.

Looking back now, I realize that was my first major reset. All the things I used to take for granted — a salary at the end of the month, a holiday allowance, job security — were suddenly gone. I literally had to start from scratch again, but I have never regretted it for one moment.

The coronavirus crisis gives me another opportunity to start afresh. But what if we all decide to begin 2022 by pressing 'reset' and starting with a clean sheet? Incidentally, you don't need a crisis for this; you can instigate a reset whenever you want. But a life-changing event such as a pandemic can help you take a step back and look at what is wrong with your life.

Of course we humans can't simply be returned to the factory settings as is the case with a computer or smartphone. We always keep our past experiences. I based my company's services on my research into resilience, for instance. If I should ever decide on another professional reset (which is quite likely as my hobby is interior design, but more on that later), then I will be able to draw on my experience of running a business and creating a brand.

Moreover, a human reset is not a brief, time-limited event; it is a process in which you are continually re-evaluating and improving the situation. And unlike the Great Reset that Klaus Schwab announced at the World Economic Forum in June 2020, my reset is not restricted to the happy few. I will consider this reset at the individual, most tangible level in the first instance, and only then look at the implications for schools, businesses and politicians. Anyone with an open mindset can learn something here. This book aims to be relevant and practical.

CHAPTER 2

IT DEPENDS HOW YOU LOOK AT IT

WHY A CRISIS IS ALWAYS AN OPPORTUNITY TOO

"The mental impact of the lockdown is much greater than that of the virus," I claimed confidently in April 2020 in an interview with a Belgian newspaper. I really did believe this when the pandemic started, and research confirmed my gut feeling. For example, 31 per cent of the respondents in a survey in the US at the end of June 2020 reported symptoms of anxiety and depression, almost twice as many as before the pandemic. At that point, the crisis looked as if it was having a huge negative impact on our mental wellbeing — even though we did not then realize how long it would last.

Recent figures give a more nuanced picture. In the Netherlands, the proportion of people in poor mental health was the same in 2020 as in the four previous years, at 12 per cent of the population. A study published in the *Lancet* showed that suicide rates even fell in some countries during the first few months of the pandemic. It is not yet known why this happened, neither do we know yet whether this effect will be sustained but in my view this shows clearly that the mental benefits of the crisis can compete with the downsides. It may sound weird to say so, but the crisis has done a lot of good for our mental wellbeing. Precisely because the coronavirus crisis has lasted so long, many people have managed to find a new equilibrium. "More time for my family"; "healthier eating habits that have helped me finally get a grip on my eating disorder"; "better able to concentrate than in our open-plan office". Whenever I do an online session for a company and ask employees about the positive effects of the crisis, I am flooded by positive messages. The pandemic was not just challenging for our mental wellbeing, it was also a huge opportunity and we have gradually begun to realize this.

It is not my intention in this book to belittle the experiences of the many people who have had a very tough time over the past months. COVID-19 was far from the great equalizer that it was claimed to be at the start of the crisis. Some people ended up in poverty, lost relatives or struggled with the effects of long Covid. We may have all been in the same storm, but we were not all in the same boat. The social isolation, for instance, had much greater consequences for some groups than others. The elderly were less able to use digital means of communication than younger generations, which made them more vulnerable. Health workers who had to deal with the impact of the pandemic on a daily basis or were required to make ethical choices also ran a bigger risk of adverse mental effects.

I personally was one of the privileged, like many people in my circle. I have privileges that made the experience much more bearable: my daughters, meaningful work, a warm network and space. I am fully aware of that. If your family are living on top of one another and don't have enough money to make ends meet, that has a gigantic impact that is difficult for me to imagine. If you belong to that group, your resilience is being seriously challenged. Sometimes you see that it is precisely those people who are exceptionally resilient, although that is far from a foregone conclusion. As Professor Patrick Luyten wrote in an opinion piece, "Try being resilient during the COVID-19 pandemic if you live in a context characterized by poverty, violence, neglect and hopelessness, with almost nobody who can give you a nudge in the right direction. It's a lot easier in a nice detached house with its own garden." Even so, there are plenty of occupants of 'detached houses with gardens' who wallowed in misery and impotence.

We can't do much about our genes, upbringing or circumstances. But the final deciding factor is our mindset. Or as Professor

Lieven Annemans puts it, “Even someone who has nothing to complain about can still be unhappy.” I am sorry to say that in the past year I saw people with a fixed mindset, a lack of meta-awareness and a tendency to see themselves as the underdog getting stuck in a negative spiral. They felt lonely but didn’t do enough to reach out to others. They reacted despondently to every new measure and as a consequence forgot what was still possible. The way they dealt with the virus gave them stress and burnout symptoms. They slept poorly, which only increased their pessimistic thoughts.

On the other hand, the people who focused on the things they could control and did not see the pandemic as something that simply happened to them were often much better able to cope with the crisis. The same applied to the people who adopted a positive explanatory style and made the best of it rather than giving up because “everything has gone to pot anyway”. If you believe you take control and your fate doesn’t depend entirely on your boss or society at large, you are much more likely to take ownership of the situation and make the most of it. The good news is that you can learn this!

Indeed, whether you can get anything out of this book doesn’t depend on your circumstances so much as on your mindset. If you are prepared to change, then I can assure you this book will be more than a drop in the ocean. Perhaps you find it difficult to spot the silver linings of COVID-19. And yet you may have already learned quite a few positive lessons and new habits, whether consciously or unconsciously. I will run through some of them for you.

Never waste a good crisis

I have long been convinced that a crisis can be a time of strength. You may think it is just a cliché from rags-to-riches films and novels, but scientific research shows that exceptionally successful people have often had to overcome serious obstacles on their road to success. The British psychologist John Nicholson conducted in-depth interviews to find the common denominator among highly successful people. The result? It turned out that they had faced tough circumstances early on in their lives and had to fight their way to the top. So people who flourish haven't always had it easy, but they did not give up when confronted with setbacks.

The perfect example of this for me is the current US president, Joe Biden. As a young senator, he lost his wife Emilia and daughter in a traffic accident. His two sons gave him the strength to keep going. But then his eldest son, Beau, passed away at the age of 46 from a brain tumour. Hunter, the younger son, struggled for years with severe addiction to alcohol and drugs. Yet these personal tragedies did not stop Joe Biden from climbing to become president of the United States. In my opinion, it is no coincidence that he remained calm and firm during the election campaign while the then president Donald Trump did everything he could to break Biden. Life had prepared him for it.

I too have experienced some crises in my life — as you will be able to read in later chapters. It is precisely that experience that has made me strong. I know I will always be able to keep going and that I can be flexible. I gained immense confidence in myself as a result. Whatever crisis comes my way, I can be sure I will cope.

Even when I feel miserable, I always think I'll get there in the end. In fact, I always believe things will get better. A lot better.

In psychology, we use the concept of post-traumatic growth, the personal growth some people experience after going through a tough period. I mentioned earlier that many of the survivors of the *Herald of Free Enterprise* shipwreck in 1987 actually felt better afterwards. They were able to enjoy the little things in life more and worried less about unimportant matters.

That research is precisely why, as a psychologist, I was regularly rubbing my hands with glee during the coronavirus crisis. While I initially feared that the mental impact of the crisis would be worse than that of the virus itself, I gradually started to realize what an amazing opportunity lay hidden within this collective trauma. It may sound strange and I certainly intend no disrespect for the health workers who are now running on empty or the many relatives of people who died from COVID-19, but if I'm honest I would not have wanted to miss this period.

The realization that we could use this crisis as a catalyst for change came to me in September 2020. Just when we thought COVID-19 was over — I was already giving talks to live audiences in the Netherlands — stricter measures had to be reintroduced. The sprint we thought we were in suddenly turned out to be a marathon. And the finish line kept being moved further away. The duration and impact of the crisis on nearly all fronts made me realize that the coronavirus would be decisive for us as a society and for future generations. Hybrid work would be here to stay and we would not be prepared to return to the rat race of the past. We would no longer put up with a life in which we spend most of the day at work, followed by the commute home in traffic jams, with just about enough time at the end of the day to give our kids a quick goodnight kiss.

CLOSING DOORS

Seeing a crisis as an opportunity for transformation and growth does not mean disregarding the challenges. Re-evaluating a situation from a different, more positive perspective – termed cognitive reappraisal – should not become a denial of the negative emotions. Therapists should also not try to turn negative emotions into something positive straight away, said motivation psychologist Maarten Vansteenkiste in the 'Mental Equilibrium in Young People' webinar organized by Driven by Health. "If you do that, you meet with resistance because you are failing to recognize the person's efforts. You are completely disregarding their emotional experience."

It is quite all right to be exasperated about the situation. You don't need to suppress your anger and distress or try to forget them as soon as possible. After all, you can only let go of your anger and distress, reducing their power over you, once you have acknowledged those feelings. This is known as the acceptance paradox. You can only change and grow once you have accepted yourself as you are and acknowledged your problems. This conclusion was reached by the influential American psychologist Carl Rogers. People who get stuck time and again in their change process often think they are simply not capable of changing anything. Wrong, said Rogers. They can change things but the real problem is that they don't come clean with themselves.

Mourning rituals and sites of remembrance can help create room for collective grief and acceptance. That is also the case for this pandemic. Some examples are the empty body bags with the national flag on the beach at Rio de Janeiro, or the red hearts on a wall in London commemorating coronavirus victims. In your own life too, a gesture or ritual can help you put the challenges of the coronavirus crisis behind you. "It is always important to know when something has reached its end. Closing circles, shutting doors, finishing chapters...

it doesn't matter what we call it; what matters is to leave in the past those moments in life that are over," wrote Paulo Coelho. When one door closes, another one opens, as the saying goes. Only then can you see the many opportunities. Because they really are out there.

Fine is suspect

""How are you?" "Fine. Busy, of course. How about you?" "Great, great." That's what we said to one another before the coronavirus crisis. It was even worse in the US, where I lived for a while. There, people often replied "fantastic" or "awesome". We may have rowed with our partner the previous day, be worried about our parents' fragile health or under huge stress, but our answer was always "fine" and that was apparently what the person asking wanted to hear. So often, instead of "How are you?" we got "Everything OK?" because people feel uncomfortable with the mere idea that someone might reply "Not so good".

But the coronavirus crisis has made "Great, great" no longer an acceptable answer. Even "Fine" sounds rather suspicious. We have all been facing mental challenges and we know that. When we were working from home *en masse*, we literally opened up our living rooms to our work colleagues. Some people saw this as the ideal opportunity to dispense with the meaningless small talk they'd always engaged in at the water cooler and to open up their hearts too. In the past, I wouldn't have bothered with such check-ins but now I take them seriously.

During one of my many video calls in lockdown with Liesbeth, a client I've known for years, I got the "Great, great" answer. I asked her immediately, "How do you manage that? Because I feel quite down today with everything looking so bleak." Liesbeth was surprised. "You, down? But you write books about resilience!" I explained to her that I sometimes have an off day when my hormones and emotions get out of control. Even though I know from experience that I will pull through in the longer term, that does not mean I am perfectly resilient every single day. If life throws me a challenge, I too can succumb to gloomy thoughts.

After I had shown my vulnerable side, the protective shield between us evaporated. My willingness to admit my own insecurities let us have a deep and open conversation. Liesbeth confessed that things were actually not great at all. Her daughter had been admitted to a psychiatric institution with suicidal thoughts and she was worried stiff.

Since then, my standard reply whenever someone asks "Everything OK?" is "Most things are OK". It is never the case that absolutely everything is OK and because I am acknowledging my vulnerability, the other person feels free to do the same. That does not mean that I tell every client all about my relationship problems; sometimes I open up about professional challenges or everyday issues like the stress of moving house or finding the right school for my children.

I'm not the only one doing this. This public vulnerability is something I have noticed everywhere. It was already a trend on social media, and in the past year we have also seen elite sportspeople such as the cyclist Tom Dumoulin, the tennis player Naomi Osaka and the gymnast Simone Biles going public about their mental health issues. I also see it as a hopeful sign that even companies with a highly rational corporate culture are starting to have that conversation. Hopefully this crisis will give us an opportunity to talk about our mental wellbeing more often. Let's make this mainstream.

Most people are decent folk

According to international studies, the learning loss that primary-school and secondary-school children have suffered during the coronavirus crisis will have permanent consequences in their education and later at work. If you have solid financial and social resources, this is a resolvable problem but children from disadvantaged backgrounds are at risk of falling by the wayside. In the long term this could lead to greater inequality and polarization. That is why I and dozens of other Flemish businesspeople committed to spending one week in 2021 teaching at a summer school. Rather than calling on the government, we decided to take action ourselves. In our Open Letter, we explained:

"The coronavirus crisis is our Second World War. Our children and grandchildren will ask us what we did to resolve the problems, repair the damage and make the world a better place. It is too easy to call on someone else to take action. Let's take action ourselves. Because together we make up society. And each of us has a duty to do their bit."

If someone had approached leading businesspeople a few years ago with the idea of teaching at a summer school, the reaction might well have been less enthusiastic. But as Rutger Bregman, the historian and author of *Human kind: A Hopeful History*, knows, most people are decent folk and essentially want the best for their fellow human beings. This action is just one of the many spontaneous expressions of solidarity that were prompted by the coronavirus crisis. Around the world, 'shopping angels' bought groceries for the most vulnerable, neighbours posted notes in one another's letterboxes offering help, cakes were delivered to hospitals for health workers and people donated money to save their favourite restaurant, bar or shop.

Covid reminded everyone of what really matters in life. We discovered we are social creatures who need to connect with others. Money doesn't make us happy. That yearning for contact led people to show real solidarity *en masse*; this was the ultimate confirmation for me that humans are essentially decent beings. Or as Oxfam wrote in an opinion piece: "2020 will go on record as the year in which we brought the economy to a standstill in order to save lives. We can be proud of this because it shows we are social, empathic beings. We were prepared to make unprecedented sacrifices, both individually and collectively, to flatten the curve of infections, hospital admissions, intensive care treatments and deaths."

It is possible

If someone had predicted on 1 January 2020 that we would spend months working from home, that we would be home-schooling our children and that we would not be able to see our friends or family for long stretches, no one would have believed them. We would probably have said this was unrealistic and impossible. We would never be able to look after our children without the help of their grandparents, we would never be able to run our companies without face-to-face meetings and we would never be able to restrict our wedding guest list to ten invites.

Now we know all these things are possible. In relatively short order, we were able to change everything about our lives and assumptions. Knowing that should give you self-confidence. If we can manage that, what else could we do? Of course we don't need to wait for the next crisis to transform our lives. Bring it on!

My hairdresser, for example, announced that she would be closing the shop for two months in the summer of 2021 as she would be doing the hairstyles for an international show in Valencia. "A chance of a lifetime!" She would never have dared do that before the coronavirus crisis. "I couldn't close my hairdresser's for two months. I'm young and I've got a business to run. Where would my regular customers go?" After her shop had been closed for months anyway, she was prepared to take that step. "I survived the lockdown and apparently so did my customers' hair. So a scheduled closure of two months will be OK too. Anyway, I realize I need to seize this opportunity now, as life is so unpredictable."

How often in the past did we have a great idea that we never put into practice because we thought we were too busy or the time wasn't right? How often did we sabotage ourselves with these thoughts? I predict that we will be less inclined to say "I can't do that" in future, and more inclined to quote Pippi Longstocking: "I've never tried that before, so I think I should definitely be able to do it." My expectation is that we will feel less impotent as a result and our self-efficacy — our confidence that we can achieve our goals — will increase. Isn't it wonderful how this seismic shift has set things in motion that we would never have imagined possible!

Fortunately the crisis went on long enough

Many people are hoping that they will be able to keep up their healthy lunches after the coronavirus crisis ends, that they will still be planning walks with friends and that they will build in enough breathing space in their diaries. However, experience with New Year's resolutions has made many fear these aspirations may not last either. Why would we keep our resolutions this time when we usually fail? Yet there are enough reasons to think this time will be different.

When you remember that it takes an average of 66 days to learn a new habit, you will realize how lucky we have been that the crisis went on so long. Our good resolutions have had over a year to take root. That is very different to starting a fitness regime on 1 January based purely on willpower and giving up two weeks later. When you have spent over a year walking everywhere, the car will no longer be your default option for short distances. After spending the entire pandemic cooking healthy food, you will know the recipes like the back of your hand.

"But what about the traffic jams, Elke? Even when working from home was still obligatory, congestion started to increase again as if there had never been any Covid." It is true that we have gone back to bad old habits to a certain extent: even in the spring of 2021, there were already a lot more people on the roads. But I am convinced that plenty of the good habits we developed will survive as well. After all, we experienced new things that we will never want to give up.

For example, in the summer of 2021, I saw a shift towards more outdoor activities. The outdoor seating at cafes and restaurants was extended (even after we were allowed to eat inside), outdoor gyms became booming business and numerous art exhibitions were set up in nature. And the people who decided on a staycation demonstrated a preference for activities such as hiking and cycling in the countryside rather than visiting urban cultural centres. Spending more time outdoors is good for our wellbeing. Hopefully that is a development that is here to stay.

I also believe spending more time with the family is a permanent shift. I can't imagine we will want to give that up and if we do, the kids will protest. They too are used to this new normal. That means people will start setting limits to protect private time. It is just one of the reasons why the return to the office will not necessarily go smoothly in a lot of companies. More about that later.

Great: we aren't in control

If the coronavirus has taught us one thing, it is that we cannot influence the world around us. The world cannot be engineered to suit us, even if we had wanted that in 2021. Control is for the current generations what freedom was for the hippies in the 1960s, said philosopher and psychiatrist Damiaan Denys in an interview in *New Scientist*. "Control has become a virtue. If you ask someone how they are doing, they say, 'Fine, everything's under control!' With our smartphones and our insurance policies: we want to know constantly exactly where we are going, how much money we have in the bank and what we can expect. The need for control is extreme." When a virus brought the world to its knees, the idea that everything can be controlled was shown to be an illusion. Many people found that hard to accept.

And yet that lack of control is a blessing, says Denys, for that limitation is a source of creativity — as artists know all too well. Take the classic block that artists experience when they are given free rein. But give them a context and a list of restrictions and their creative juices start flowing. "I don't find instructions limiting — quite the opposite," I read in an interview with the illustrator Gerda Dendooven. "I actually like going as far as I can within a predefined framework. If anything is allowed, you start freewheeling and I often find that paralysing."

That even extreme restrictions can produce outstanding art was demonstrated by Ernest Hemingway with his "For Sale, Baby Shoes, Never Worn". Legend has it that this example of flash fiction was the result of a bet between Hemingway and a bar owner in the Florida Keys. The barman claimed it would be impossible for Hemingway to write a story in just six words with as much depth as his books. Hemingway won the bet with his advertisement for baby shoes. Whether Hemingway really was the author is debatable but the six-word story has become a literary genre in its own right.

In short, we don't have much control over the world around us but that is not a problem. What we can control are our own brains. During the pandemic, we all discovered how resilient we are, depending on whether we feed our inner underdog or top dog. We discovered at first hand that off days don't brighten up if we wallow in them, and that worrying doesn't stop if we isolate ourselves. What is more, when all the extraneous stuff in our lives was removed, we were able to see quite clearly what exactly gave us energy and what sucked the life out of us. Minor actions could have a major impact on a day or a week. I found out that if I set my alarm 15 minutes earlier, I no longer get stressed about taking the children to school on time. If I go for a walk during my lunch break, I am much less likely to have a dip in the afternoon.

Finally there's a problem needs solving

Before the pandemic, people in the West were living "like firefighters without fire", according to the Israeli thinker Yuval Noah Harari. We were incredibly spoilt. Apart from a few private problems, most of us have hardly experienced any really tough times, said Damiaan Denys when he was interviewed about a game show in which he investigates why it is that the Netherlands consistently ranks among the happiest countries in global lists while so many individual people there feel discontented. "We live in a very strange society in which happiness has become a goal in its own right. In the past, we were too busy making sure we had enough to eat and drink for that." According to Denys, the result is that we have forgotten how to make room for normal suffering.

I agree. Because we have not had to exercise our resilience muscle much, we obsessed about the coronavirus pandemic, whereas a hundred years ago, this crisis might have been just a minor blip in history. Covid took us all out of our comfort zone. But that means we were all gifted an opportunity to grow. Once you have encountered a situation that feels stressful, you will recognize that feeling the next time. New neural pathways have been created. You will know immediately that you are capable of dealing with the challenging situation and will feel more confident and less stressed as a result. But if you routinely avoid tricky situations, you are depriving yourself of the opportunity to discover your inner strength.

That is why I consider the pandemic to be a transformation. We have been transformed as humans, as families, as teams and as citizens. Many people quit the rat race, started eating more healthily and focused more on what really matters in life. I hope that as individuals and as society at large we will grow thanks to this experience.

Incidentally, it is good to know that this is not an either/or case: it's not either post-traumatic stress or post-traumatic growth. Various studies even suggest that some post-traumatic stress actually boosts growth. So people can experience both growth *and* trauma-related symptoms. They can grow and suffer or feel grief at the same time.

WHAT IF YOU REALLY CAN'T SEE THE SILVER LININGS?

Among the mountain of positive messages I get when I do sessions for companies, there is regularly also one from someone who can't see any silver linings and has got nothing positive at all out of the crisis.

Perhaps you are one such person, or this was your response to a previous crisis. Perhaps you see the cracks, but not the light that gets in. In such a situation, what works well is to ask yourself critical questions about your thoughts – a technique from the Appreciative Inquiry approach. For example, I recently caught myself saying I was having an off day. Instead of fixating on that, I asked myself some questions. "Was it really such a bad day, or was that just my impression? Did things happen today that I'm grateful for?" I soon discovered my alleged off day had also had some bright spots. Putting my meta-awareness to work let me radically change my assessment.

This process of critically asking myself questions has become a thoroughly embedded reflex for me but if you are not yet at that stage, a useful method is to keep a gratitude diary in which you note down three things you are grateful for every day. If you keep this up, you will discover that you automatically start to notice the light through the cracks.

We can start with a lovely clean sheet

In June 2021, my newly formed family and I moved house to the countryside. Our new home had a perfectly functional kitchen. Our relatives thought we could easily manage with the existing kitchen for a few more years but I decided it had to go immediately. Our relatives couldn't understand why but I didn't waver. I knew that if I was going to have to work in that kitchen for the next few years, I would constantly be irritated. I am quite tall and the worktops were simply too low. That kitchen would result in me losing time and energy. Moreover, I could already foresee the appliances needing to be replaced one after another. So when we did come to replace the kitchen in five years' time, we would be tempted to incorporate that recently purchased oven and dishwasher in the new kitchen, meaning I would never have a completely new, streamlined kitchen. It would always be a mishmash. So I stuck to my guns and replaced the kitchen immediately. It took trouble and courage: all that money, all that hassle. But I have never regretted the result for one moment.

It might sound strange but my kitchen reset has some similarities with the transformation we are all undergoing thanks to Covid. Because we temporarily lost everything during the crisis — our hobbies, friends and family, the commute to the office — we gained the opportunity to rebuild our lives from scratch. We could choose to start playing tennis once a week again, but scrap the monthly visits to the hairdresser. We could resume our picnics with a friend but no longer spend hours in the kitchen preparing food for a dinner party. It is much simpler to rebuild your life starting with a clean sheet than to tinker with it when you have a full diary.

You can compare this to what happened after the Second World War. The Belgian economy was able to recover relatively quickly as key components of the infrastructure such as the railways were largely intact. As a result, Belgian companies could soon resume normal operations. In the Netherlands and Germany, the infrastructure had suffered far more damage and so recovery took longer. However, five years later the roles were reversed. By then Belgium had outdated infrastructure whereas Germany and the Netherlands were flourishing thanks to their modern, efficient ports and railways.

The Dutch historian Jan Romein called this the handicap of a head start versus the stimulus from coming from behind. If I had kept the old kitchen, I would have been able to cook fresh, healthy meals in the first few weeks after the move instead of having to live off takeaways. But I might not have felt encouraged to try out new recipes or improve my culinary skills in the months and years that followed if I was stuck with that old kitchen. Taking out the kitchen and replacing it cost us a few weeks of making do but I could cook much faster and better in the new one than would ever have been possible in the old one. Want to bet our post-Covid reset will be similar?

HYBRID HEALTHCARE

"For years we were pregnant with digital care. That baby has finally been delivered thanks to the crisis, with an emergency caesarean," says Lucien Engelen, CEO of Transform.Health. The coronavirus crisis gave online consultations with doctors and psychologists the shot in the arm that they needed. At first, consultations moved online because of the Covid restrictions but this trend looks here to stay. The following step was apps that let you make a digital appointment with a qualified physician wherever you happen to be physically. That gives me hope, not just for physical healthcare but also for mental healthcare.

Not only have online therapies been proven to work (including for anxiety disorders, social phobias and mild to moderate depression) but digital consultations also have some important advantages. Firstly, you don't have to travel anywhere. It is hardly surprising that the pioneer in online therapy is Australia, a country where distances are huge. And while it is easier to make weekly visits to the psychologist in more densely populated countries, a half-hour trip can still be difficult to fit into our busy lives and put us off seeking help. Online therapy in your native language can also bring relief to expats and visitors who go through an emotional crisis in a foreign country.

Moreover, online therapy can be less intimidating emotionally. In the United States, where people have been using online therapy websites for longer, users report less shame and say they feel safer. The reluctance to consult a psychologist is a widespread phenomenon and means people put off seeking help, sometimes until it is too late. An accessible platform that lets you consult a psychologist from your own living room could reduce that delay.

The labour market is also a problem in the health sector, and many countries have difficulty recruiting and training enough staff. E-health applications could help resolve this issue too. Behavioural therapists, for example, could monitor patients between sessions via a coaching app that sends the patient reminders and keeps track of progress. Perhaps fewer sessions would then be needed per patient without having to compromise on quality. It also means the mental health professional is always on hand for the patient. There are also many benefits to be gained from e-health when it comes to prevention. For instance, a potential psychosis could be spotted by an app that analyses your clicks – provided this is done with respect for privacy, of course.

All this sounds fantastic, but I am not advocating the complete digitalization of our health services. As in education and business, I believe in a hybrid approach in which face-to-face consultations with a psychologist or doctor are intermixed with digital sessions or monitoring using e-health applications. "E-health will not replace in-person care," says Sebastiaan Blok, head of research at the Dutch cardiology care network CCN. "Just as music streaming services won't replace concert halls." Yet he still believes e-health is inevitable. "We have a new generation that no longer finds it obvious that you take a day off and travel a long way for a health check and a doctor's appointment. Now we are all banking and booking our holidays online, healthcare will increasingly be delivered digitally too. We can also draw lessons for digital healthcare from the digitalization that is taking place in society more broadly: (1) I can listen to as much music as I want on Spotify for a monthly subscription; (2) listening to Spotify lets me know what music I want to experience live; (3) the live performance is always better, but listening online is mostly good enough."

"They are us"

"We often feel angry because we haven't been acknowledged. That is usually coupled with sadness — sadness about the loss of a certain way of life or a cherished hope. Politicians could regain the public's confidence by recognizing that sadness." These are the words of the philosopher Tinneke Beeckman in the magazine *Psychologies*. This is her answer to the question of why so many people — the Gilets Jaunes, the anti-vax protesters, the young climate campaigners — are so angry with the authorities.

She is right. Underlying that anger is sadness about what may well have been lost irrevocably. I have also become more willing to get angry since I became a mother. Because what kind of a world will my children inherit, with threats of viruses, fake news and global warming? Unfortunately, I see little sign of empathy for this sadness from the authorities. On the contrary, politicians often react to the violent emotions of the people, whether on the left or the right, with a certain degree of disdain. In 2016, Hillary Clinton called the discontented Americans who supported Trump "a basket of deplorables". If you make such a disparaging statement, you should not be surprised that Trump went on to win the election. Such remarks only exacerbate the people's anger.

One politician who has demonstrated that strong leadership and empathy can go together perfectly well is New Zealand's prime minister, Jacinda Ardern. Her words in reference to the Muslim community after the attacks in Christchurch have become famous: "They are us". Those words of reconciliation were accompanied by decisive measures to tighten the gun laws. Ardern adopted an exceptionally rigorous approach to the pandemic too, but because she continually stressed that people needed to be kind to one another, she still managed to get everyone to support her strict policies. She would often spend her evenings answering questions from the general public on Facebook Lives from her living room. Arden got her "team of five million" through the crisis by using empathy. People obeyed the measures and the number of casualties was kept low.

I thought of Jacinda Ardern when a good friend of mine complained in spring 2021 that B., a school friend of hers, did not want to get vaccinated. My friend was angry. How could B. believe those conspiracy theories? She was so irritated that she considered temporarily breaking contact with B. At first, I couldn't think how to calm my friend down, but then I remembered Ardern's words "They are us". I said soothingly to my friend, "B. and you go a long way back. You care so much about each other but you don't agree on this particular matter. That is not a problem as long as you can still respect one another." My friend said she would think about it. A week later, I heard she and B. were going to meet up again for a coffee. "It was the first time we had had such a fundamental difference of opinion," said my friend. "But we talked, and it's a relief to find that we respect one another enough to overcome our differences."

The coronavirus crisis and the policies introduced to tackle it led to more ethical discussions than is normally the case. There were couples where one partner was much laxer with the rules than the other. There were companies where the vaccinated thought the unvaccinated posed a danger to everyone. There were families where the dilemma of whether to celebrate Christmas together caused rows for weeks. Did this inevitably lead to a rupture? I very much doubt it. Of course there are exceptions, but I suspect most people were able to maintain the contact despite the differences of opinion. Perhaps we will demonstrate more respect in future for Uncle Josh's aberrant political beliefs and cousin Mary's toe-curling opinions?

Empathy has a limited shelf life... but you can extend it

July 2021. After the severe flooding in Belgium, 14,000 people immediately offered their services as volunteers on the Red Cross website. The images of the floods had made a deep impression. There had been dozens of fatalities and many houses had become uninhabitable. There was an urgent need for aid and people were ready to help.

So there was general indignation when the Red Cross announced in the days that followed that it did not need any voluntary helpers as yet. One week later, only 144 volunteers had been put to work. The official message was that the Red Cross wanted to coordinate the effort, match the need for aid with the aid workers and brief the volunteers on safety. This meant that the town of Pepinster saw the Israeli Red Cross marching through the streets before the Belgian Red Cross arrived.

What a contrast with spontaneous initiatives from the public such as Aidehulp 14-17, in which professionals such as electricians and builders offered to help local people. Even lawyers offered their services to people affected by the floods who wanted to submit a damage claim. And lots of people turned up with vans, cleaning equipment and food trucks. They ignored the Red Cross's assessment that you can't send 'inexperienced' volunteers to a disaster area to help clear out cellars, remove ravaged household goods and hand out hot meals.

These gestures of solidarity were incredibly valuable, not just in practical terms but also because of their psychological effect.

Sufferers felt buoyed by the fact that so many strangers wanted to help them — they did not have to face this alone. What did it matter if not every mop was used efficiently and not every van packed expertly? The many helping hands alleviated the misery and strengthened the sense of community. The helpers in turn felt more in control over the situation: they did not have to look on powerlessly as thousands of people were left homeless.

What a missed opportunity for the Red Cross, which was supposed to be coordinating the effort! If they had been better able to channel the large number of volunteers from the start, the aid actions might well have been better coordinated. They would also have been able to deploy the voluntary helpers just when their levels of empathy were at their peak; those volunteers would then have been permanently committed to the Red Cross.

After all, empathy has its own shelf life. You may well have experienced how after a while you become immune to images of a disaster. Or if the Red Cross only contacts you to ask for your help one month after the floods, that you are no longer so interested. But if you become involved in a charitable cause at the point when your empathy is greatest, you feel committed and this lets you extend your empathy. The same happens if you delve into a particular issue and search for background articles that discuss the various nuances of that crisis. But if your news consumption remains superficial, the steady stream of images and stories soon blurs into one undifferentiated mass. That is why I avoid reading coronavirus blogs on news websites. After a while I can no longer process those rapid updates: they go in one ear and out the other. I prefer to read just a few longer articles at the weekend. I find that I am more engaged with the issue then than if I see all the news flashes appearing every day.

It will be all right in the end (and better than ever)

""If we don't keep to the measures, the health service won't be able to cope and patients will end up dying in the corridors." Politicians and virologists regularly issued warnings like these over the past year in an effort to keep us in line. If you urgently want to change people's behaviour, sowing fear is one possible strategy. At the start of the pandemic, when no one seemed to realize how serious it was, the population was jolted awake with a message designed to frighten them. That was thought to be the only way to make imposing a sudden, stringent lockdown possible. I admit I too needed a wake-up call before I took the situation seriously. However, while it is fine to raise awareness, there was no need to instigate fear in that way. After all, our brains do strange things under extreme stress. We start stockpiling toilet rolls, even though there was no rational reason why there might be a shortage of toilet rolls.

A frightening message is even more counterproductive in the longer term. If people feel anxious, they try to get rid of that feeling. They stick their heads in the sand. That is precisely why people eventually start to ignore the confrontational photos of smokers' lungs on cigarette packets. What is more, fear is polarizing. When we are scared, we are less likely to help others: it is every man for himself. That is also why I am not a fan of the French president Macron's announcement that "We are at war".

Of course, when you are in a crisis, you don't want to play down or underestimate the danger. But it is perfectly possible to make people aware of the danger without scaremongering. Some virologists remained calm throughout and were crystal clear in their communication. They offered people hope, which is crucial in a long-lasting crisis like COVID-19.

Hence my call for more inspiring, enthusiastic messages and more positive news items. That works! Focusing on the doom and gloom only leads to fatalism, while focusing on progress leads to positive change. That applies to our private lives and work too. Entrepreneurs who responded to the pandemic with innovations and were prepared to think outside the box were able to transform some sectors, perhaps for good. It's so handy that nowadays you can pay for everything with your smartphone and that you can put in an order at a restaurant via a QR code. And it's so inspirational to now be able to attend an international conference in my discipline online while sitting at home. The way that Japan organized the Olympic Games in the summer of 2021 was incredibly impressive. For a moment it looked as if the doomsayers who were predicting a new wave of infections would be proved right and the Games would be postponed once again. But the optimists seized the opportunity to experiment with technological innovation. Potentially risky contacts between the athletes and the local population were minimized by transporting the athletes in self-driving vans, while robots picked up the discus and tennis balls. The athletes and their entourage could use contactless check-ins everywhere thanks to facial recognition. Thanks to the optimists, the Japanese Olympic Games will go down in history as the most technologically advanced to date and may well act as a catalyst for the transport, robots and safety protocols of the future. Perhaps the event will speed up change...

"WE WILL MEET AGAIN"

24 April 2020, 10 pm. The prime minister Sophie Wilmès addressed the Belgian people. She explained the exit strategy – how Belgium would phase out the coronavirus control measures – using a PowerPoint presentation. The font on the slides was so small that the text was illegible, the phased structure was sloppy and the explanation lengthy, dry and tedious.

Wilmès' PowerPoint presentation may well have been comprehensive, but she failed to achieve her objective. She did not get her message across. Half the country had switched off before she even got to the end, and gone outside to watch Elon Musk's Starlink train cross the skies. That appealed more to the imagination.

How different Ghana's president, Nana Akufo-Addo, sounded a few weeks earlier with his statement: "We know how to bring the economy back to life. What we do not know is how to bring people back to life." This message encapsulated the situation: it was clear, catchy, easy to remember and made a link with the 'why'.

A catchy message can help maintain a focus. Such slogans may be populist or facile but I find them far more inspiring than the words of prime minister Wilmès. Even 94-year-old Queen Elizabeth II in the UK did better: "We will be with our friends again; we will be with our families again; we will meet again." She touched the hearts of the British people.

When I told my team about my pandemic policy for Better Minds at Work, I tried to do the same. Instead of focusing on rules, measures, dots and commas, I summarized everything with a single notion: bouncing forward. How could we emerge from the crisis stronger than ever, as staff and as a company? That was the question I asked myself with every decision I took. That was the question I wanted my employees to ask themselves when I invited them to think about their and our future. Everything else followed from that.

The end of "must" as the driving force

"Don't give up." "Use your common sense." "The new variant is 30% more contagious, so watch out." These are not very motivating messages. Why exactly do you need to be so cautious? What does "30% more contagious" mean precisely? What is the actual risk?

Motivation psychologist Maarten Vansteenkiste soon realized that this kind of communication was not going to have the desired effect. In collaboration with researchers at Finnish and Australian universities, he studied how this could be improved. In January 2021, the international research team published thirteen communication principles based on the theory of self-determination and designed to promote voluntary compliance with the rules. After all, many of the measures depended on our personal commitment: the government couldn't exactly monitor how often we were washing our hands. Voluntary compliance with the rules encourages ownership too. An intrinsically motivated population is more resilient than a population that is forced to comply with measures through various control mechanisms.

The first set of guidelines is all about autonomy. Explain what the effect of a measure is, appeal to people's sense of responsibility, show that you trust them and don't pressurize them by using the word 'must'. Furthermore, emphasize universal norms and values — protecting the weak — and show what is still possible under the current restrictions.

The second set focuses on supporting competences. Give concrete instructions and formulate shared objectives with clear, unambiguous parameters that are monitored constantly. Give feedback, such as statistics showing how certain measures have helped flatten the curve. Identify possible obstacles and present ideas about how to tackle them.

The final set of guidelines deals with trust. Acknowledge the difficulties caused by the measures, emphasize that we are all affected, be transparent, including about the potential risks, use scientists and people who have positions of trust in certain social groups to get the message across, and appeal to people's decency and willingness to help others.

If you keep to these guidelines in your communication, you will find people become intrinsically motivated to stick to the measures. That means you don't need to deploy drones to see whether someone has holed up in their holiday home, or have the police checking whether cafe tables are 1.5 metres apart, or visiting people's homes to check they are keeping to the quarantine rules. "That stops it being a must," says Vansteenkiste. "If you can get people intrinsically motivated, it costs less energy to stick to the rules."

Note that those guidelines were published in January 2021. The underlying theory — the ABC model of self-determination based on autonomy, belonging and competence — dates back to the mid-1980s. So did all politicians adopt a brain-friendly approach to their communication? That is not the impression I got. You may well have felt yourself that you were more motivated after some government addresses than after others. Why not do your own test? Think back to a time when you didn't agree at all with the measures (or supported them fulsomely) and see how the communication compares with the thirteen-point checklist. Illuminating, isn't it?

That is why I am now going to put the ball in business leaders' court. Clearly, these principles apply equally well to companies, for example when rolling out a policy for hybrid office work. Here too, everyone would benefit if the abovementioned guidelines on autonomy, competence support and trust were implemented. I discuss this in more detail in Chapter 5.

You can restore trust

We live in a post-truth world and our trust in our politicians is at an all-time low. No other profession is as mistrusted as politicians; even second-hand car dealers score better. That mistrust is not always justified. Politicians just have to make one false step and the opposition pounces on it and paints the culprit as a villain. It is often said that trust is hard to gain and easy to lose.

Politicians have been walking a precariously thin tightrope in the past few months. Trust had to be restored if policymakers were to avoid the tightrope snapping. But how do you restore trust? How do you generate confidence? By being honest and showing your vulnerable side. This is not news, neither to us nor to our politicians. In theory. Because you can often get a different impression in practice, with promises that keep being changed and measures that were retained much longer than had originally been announced.

If you promise something, you have to keep that promise. Try making a promise and then breaking it as a parent or employer. If I can't be sure there is an ice cream parlour at the end of a walk, I won't promise my daughters an ice cream. If I don't know whether there will be enough cash in the company's account, I won't promise my staff bonuses. People will only have confidence that things will end well in the long term if you consistently keep your promises. Only then will they be able to use their willpower to keep going.

Research shows that children whose parents regularly make promises that they don't keep, change their opinions or make threats that they never carry out will eventually stop believing in the principle of delayed rewards. They opt for instant happiness because they have no faith in the real reward that is supposed to come later. As a result, they develop weaker willpower and self-discipline. Children whose parents do keep their promises, on the other hand, learn that effort is rewarded. This motivates them to exercise more self-discipline and willpower.

We adults are no different from those children. If the measures keep changing, we lose confidence in them. Sometimes, different politicians in the same government came out of the same meeting to give radically different messages. A far more common problem was the lack of consistency in the rules. For example, in the summer of 2021 I spent a week in the Dutch seaside resort of Cadzand on the border with Belgium. When I went to the supermarket, there was complete freedom. In Knokke, a Belgian town almost next door, there were far more rules. Yet at that point the infection rates in Belgium were much lower than in the Netherlands. So I avoided the busy supermarket in Cadzand because I didn't trust the coronavirus approach. But it did make me think. If the measures are so arbitrary, why should I trust them?

While I pondered this question, I failed to notice that my daughters had now spent far too long on the iPad. I asked them to put the tablet away as we had agreed they were not allowed to watch videos in the morning. "But Mum," they said, "Granny and Grandad let us do that." As I heard myself tell them that I have different rules from their grandparents, I realized that my iPad policy was just as arbitrary as the supermarket rules. What was the underlying logic of them being allowed to use the iPad in the morning on some days, but not on others? Time to make my iPad policy less random. I explained to them that I prefer not to have them watching television so early in the day when they are still full of energy. The morning is the ideal time to exercise or be creative rather than filling their heads with stimuli. This was allowed at their grandparents because I see the time they spend there as relaxation. It wouldn't be that bad if they occasionally played with the iPad in the mornings but it would be a waste of all that energy if they did it every morning.

By making my iPad policy logical rather than arbitrary, I restored my daughters' trust. There were no more arguments about iPads that summer. Trust in the Belgian government also seemed to bounce back that summer. The enthusiasm generated by the successful Belgian vaccination campaign led to a turnaround. All you need is a positive message and actions that match your words!

CHAPTER 3

BUILD BACK BETTER

HOW TO TAKE CONTROL OF YOUR OWN LIFE

First aid for your brain in crisis times

Once you see the crisis as an opportunity for growth and change, you probably can't wait to reshape your life to fit your wishes. To be free to set the course you want, you need a certain set of tools. You will only manage a successful reset if you possess sufficient self-control, meta-awareness, focus and optimism. I already shared those four levers for enhanced resilience in the first chapter. But in times of crisis, you need some more tools in addition to these key basic skills.

HOPE-SCROLLING

Imagine yourself in the following situation: it is May 2020 and you feel a little short of breath. That scares you. Might it be the coronavirus? That would be really awkward! How are you going to manage with that work meeting? Who will look after the kids if you have to go into quarantine? And oh no, what if you passed the disease on to your parents when you waved at them in the garden?

Ten minutes later, you are more stressed than ever. Your breathing difficulties get worse and you can no longer think straight. Perhaps you should google the symptoms? And while you're at it, calculate how long the family would need to be in quarantine if one person after another gets infected. What was the situation again with long Covid? Perhaps a new, even more infectious variant has appeared.

An hour later, you are still surfing. You have now learned that an apparently healthy young woman died of the disease in Amsterdam, that virologists think we need to be more careful and that it can take up to 48 hours to get your test results.

The doom scenario takes on massive proportions in your head. The reason? You were doom-scrolling — obsessively checking online sites for bad-news updates — instead of binge-watching *Money Heist*, (during the pandemic we were binge-watching the collapse of the world in crisis). It turned out to be a very addictive vicious circle. We felt anxiety, which we then fed by searching for information that confirmed and increased our fears. That this is not good for our mental wellbeing was demonstrated by a German study that showed a clear association between exposure to news and symptoms of depression and anxiety.

So why do we still do it? Why do we stay up until the early hours of the morning checking news sites? Firstly, knowledge gives us a (false) sense of control and safety. If we are afraid, we try to find answers that let us assess whether a situation is threatening. Then there is the human fascination for bad news. We feel compelled to rubber-neck when we pass a car accident. Finally, social media platforms encourage users to spend longer on their sites and often amplify the most polarizing voices, while the traditional media weigh in too with their clickbait. Add to that the fact that many of us stopped going into the office during the pandemic, where we would have had a sanity check on our opinions from our co-workers around the water cooler, and it is hardly surprising that our doom-laden thoughts became louder and louder.

Now imagine yourself in the following situation: it is May 2020, you feel a little short of breath and you are rather scared. You pause to think: might there be some other rational explanation for my shortness of breath? Is my anxiety justified? It is quite likely that the answer to the first question will be "yes" — hay-fever season, stress at work, physical exertion, you name it — and the answer to the second question "no". End of your worries!

Self-awareness — reflecting on your thoughts with full awareness — is just one strategy for suppressing the urge to doom-scroll. You could also go looking for positive news, in other words go hope-scrolling rather than doom-scrolling. Did you know that's what a lot of Black Lives Matter activists do? In *Bearing Witness While Black: African Americans, Smartphones*, Allissa Richardson writes that many African Americans avoid doom-scrolling because they don't want to see themselves murdered time and again in the small square of their smartphone displays. Instead, they follow accounts on social media that celebrate expressions of Black joy. So rather than watching George Floyd suffocate time after time, they binge-watch Verzuz battles, virtual DJ battles that became popular during the pandemic.

PICK YOUR SWITCH-OFF

According to a Spanish online survey, the best predictor of few depressive symptoms during the lockdown was having a hobby. Before the pandemic, I often relaxed in the evenings by watching a Netflix series. Spending my evenings on the sofa in front of the TV was not a bad strategy for me at the time. I had no problem getting in my 10,000 steps a day as I rushed from one meeting to the next, and the chats during lunch, coffee breaks and networking events satisfied my need for socializing. But Netflix turned out to be far from the ideal form of relaxation after I had spent a day on my own working from home. It worked much better for me if I went outdoors, phoned a friend while going on a walk or went on a bike ride with my father.

I often explain that personal need for relaxation using the example of how flight attendants and pilots spend their free time. Because they have very different jobs while at work and are therefore using different parts of their brains, it makes sense for them to relax in different ways to let the parts of the brain they were using intensively cool off. For example, the flight attendant might prefer to relax with a book while the pilot might need some light chatter.

Since I became aware of this, I have consciously planned my free time based on my schedule for that week. On family holidays, I take non-fiction books with me about my area of expertise because I know that after a fun-packed day with my daughters on the beach, my brain will want some intellectual stimulation. But after a whole day spent writing this book, there was no better way to relax than to take my daughters swimming. In other words, your choice of switch-off is highly personal and depends on the circumstances. That is why a crisis will often need us to reassess our switch-off, if only temporarily.

A GOOD NIGHT'S SLEEP STARTS IN THE MORNING

The pandemic hasn't helped us sleep. That is not just bad for our immunity — it is estimated that one hour of extra sleep reduces your chance of a coronavirus infection by 12 per cent — but also for our resilience. Sleeping poorly gives you a sleep debt that stops your prefrontal cortex from working properly. As a result, you are less able to concentrate and find it more difficult to remain optimistic.

To improve your sleep, you first need to understand how sleep works. The flip-flop model of the Hungarian-Swiss sleep researcher Alexander A. Borbély is particularly illuminating. For high-quality sleep, our systems when asleep and when awake need to work together properly, like a light switch. "Our sleep system must be optimally activated and our awake system must be supressed," says my Better Minds at Work colleague, behavioural therapist Erik Franck. "But modern-day lifestyles mean we may carry on working and doing things until late in the evening: we put the children to bed, reply to some e-mails, practice our hobby or do a few last-minute household tasks. As a result, we end up lying awake for perhaps two hours before we finally fall asleep. Then we start worrying, which only increases the stress."

According to Borbély's model, you need to be really tired in the evening in order to switch smoothly to the sleep state. That means you need to build up the sleep drive by starting to wind down one to two hours before you go to bed: soft lighting, and no more smartphone or exercise. A familiar story. What many people don't know is that a good night's sleep starts in the morning. If you activate your waking system fully and suppress your sleep system in good time, you will feel a greater need to sleep in the evening. You can enhance this process, for example by going for a walk first thing in the morning sun. That helps our cortisol levels to peak early in the day. You don't want cortisol to peak too late because it inhibits the creation of the sleep hormone melatonin. That is why Franck recommends getting up at the same time every day, including at the weekend. After all, we sleep most deeply when our urge to sleep is at its greatest, which is about 16 hours after we woke up. If you lie in too long at the weekend, you won't be tired on Sunday evening and so you will end up lying awake for a long time and starting the week with a social jetlag.

Once you know how sleep works, there is really no reason not to change your habits and allow for the sleep and wake systems in your daily schedule. After all, improving your sleep is one of the simplest ways of becoming more resilient. Since I learned that a good night's sleep starts in the morning, I have got into the habit of going outdoors after breakfast rather than immediately starting up my laptop, and I now set the alarm clock at the weekends as well. As a result, I fall asleep almost immediately, no longer wake up in the middle of the night and feel more rested during the day. I have never been a really bad sleeper but I have now optimized the time I spend in bed. "It is actually very easy to treat sleep problems," says Franck, "as long as you are prepared to change your behaviour."

KEEP THE DOOR CLOSED

Setting priorities is energizing and increases the likelihood that you will achieve your goals. However, a well-known phenomenon when people go through a crisis is that they often drop everything, especially the fun things, in order to concentrate on the problem. They cancel all their dates with their friends because their mother is seriously ill, or they skip their exercise class because there is a reorganization at work.

I recommend doing exactly the opposite. After all, worrying doesn't get you anywhere. During the first lockdown, I went through an emotionally tough period. As I mentioned earlier, I was still sharing a home with my ex because moving house was not possible due to the Covid measures. I was also concerned about my company. I needed to perform at the highest level to get Better Minds at Work through this period. It was not easy doing that from home, with my children and former partner permanently in the vicinity. But I needed to prioritize this task. Moreover, I knew that I would get positive energy from immersing myself in this professional challenge and achieving results.

So I made sure I could work undisturbed at a time of day when my focus was at its peak — in the morning in my case. I set clear limits to when I could look after the children. Because we formalized this allocation of time, I was able to work very productively for a couple of hours every morning without feeling guilty. In the afternoons, I was there for the girls. I also went into the office now and again to present a webinar in an empty building, even though non-essential trips were banned. It was the only way I could get properly into work mode — and it was also completely safe. And when I was working from home, the door to my study remained physically and mentally closed. It was tempting to go downstairs and check everything was OK, or to join the girls as they played with their craft kits, but keeping the door shut made sure I didn't lose sight of my priorities in the morning, and in the afternoon I could give my full attention to my daughters.

EXPECT BLACK SWANS

"Since we have no idea how the world and the job market will look in 2050, we don't really know what particular skills people will need. In order to keep up with the world of 2050, you will need not merely to invent new ideas and products — you will above all need to reinvent yourself again and again," warned the Israeli thinker Yuval Noah Harari in his book *21 Lessons for the 21st Century*.

Harari could never have predicted that flexibility would already be so important in 2020, but it turned out to be a good wake-up call. The idea that you can do your current job for the rest of your working life, that your retirement will look the same as that of your parents, and that you will be able to fly anywhere as you did in the past has turned out to be an illusion. Not only is technology evolving at a breakneck pace, our understanding of what is good for us and our planet is also improving rapidly.

Given that we are well advised to consider the long term, we should be prepared to make regular switches in our lives, preferably proactively. That means lifelong learning and diversification. I will discuss this further in the chapters on work and education.

Incidentally, flexibility does not mean you need to predict what will happen. There are few certainties in life. It is not just the pandemic that has shown us this. For a long time it was assumed that all swans were white, until Willem de Vlamingh became the first European to spot a black swan in Australia in 1696. This sighting showed that the fact that no one had ever seen a black swan and they seemed so unlikely was not proof that black swans do not exist. Nowadays, the term 'black swan' is used in economics to denote an unexpected event that no one had imagined beforehand could possibly happen. Flexibility does not mean that you are fully prepared for a possible future; it means you respond resiliently to black swans and are aware that the inconceivable can always happen.

LIKE A BOXER OUTSIDE THE RING

If you train your resilience and implement a sound brain policy, there is nothing to stop you becoming a high-reliability individual, someone who takes a realistic yet optimistic view of the future and prepares mentally for the challenges ahead with an open mind.

Does that mean you need to be like a boxer in the ring, with your fists clenched, poised for the next crisis? No, I would not wish that state of alertness on anyone. We don't know what lies ahead for us. Being permanently prepared for the worst will only make you more stressed. No one can keep that up indefinitely. Boxers are only in the ring for a brief time, but they do spend all year training their boxing technique and keeping mentally strong. If you should attack a boxer at an unguarded moment, he will be ready to win the fight.

Crafting your life

If you can see the crisis as an opportunity, be sufficiently resilient and prepare your brain for times of crisis, that is when the fun starts: crafting your own life. That is not something your partner can do for you, or your family or the government or your employer. You have to do it yourself. You own your life. If your company or country sets something in motion or provides you with tools, all the better. But it is not a good idea to pin your hopes on others if you want to avoid disappointment. You are in the driver's seat. I'd like to show you some tools that can help you tackle this.

TAKE YOUR 'WHY' AS YOUR POINT OF DEPARTURE

When I turned 18, I gave a party at my house. I had been looking forward to this moment for a long time. Finally, I would be an adult. The world was my oyster. But the evening turned out very differently to how I'd expected. In addition to gift vouchers, jewellery and CDs, I also got a more morbid present: a classmate gave me his diary. I read the entries in bed after the party and discovered the diary was full of suicidal thoughts. Of course I was unable to get to sleep after that. I wanted to help the boy and spent all night composing a letter. We corresponded like this for a while and eventually he pulled through. That wasn't just down to me, of course, but it did leave me with the feeling that this was something I seemed to have a talent for.

That was why I decided to study psychology. I wanted to help other people too. That was the underlying goal that determined my choice of degree and career, my 'why'. I did indeed manage to do this at first, but the further I climbed up the academic career ladder, the less contact I had with patients. I spent most of my time writing articles. Moreover, universities are cumbersome organizations that are slow to change. That environment doesn't suit me as I like to move fast. Increasingly, my 'why' was not being addressed. That was what led me to make a switch and set up my own company, Better Minds at Work. In this organization, I can carry on helping people and if I have an idea today, it will be on the website tomorrow.

How can you discover your own 'why'? An interesting technique that is often used in careers advice is to do a scan. What gives you energy and what drains you of energy? And what do you spontaneously tend to focus on? That is your passion.

To be honest, if I were to do the scan myself today, helping other people would still be one of my 'whys' but perhaps no longer the most important one. When I was 18, I was also interested in architecture and interior design. But my teachers told me I would need to be good at maths to study that at university, and my maths skills were only mediocre. So how about psychology, I thought to myself after the diary incident? However, while at university I spent all my cash on expensive interior magazines and if I'd studied a certain number of pages in my psychology books, I rewarded myself with half an hour leafing through a magazine.

Did I not listen properly to my 'why'? Perhaps not. The older I get, the more I realize how sensitive I am to aesthetic aspects. The cover of this book was ready even before I had come up with the title. I knew which font I wanted before one letter had been written. Everything needs to look visually top-notch, from my clothes to my Prezi presentations. And the interior design of my own home is my great hobby. Everyone tells me I should do something with this talent, and I think that might well happen. I'm only 39; I still have plenty of options.

You may well find that you only discover your real 'why' later on. Dixie Dansercoer, who died in 2021, was well known in Belgium as a polar explorer but music was his first love. Later he got into windsurfing and only after that came the polar expeditions. The former *Top Gear* presenter Jeremy Clarkson, famous for his macho attitudes, surprised everyone by starting a farm at the age of 60. In *Clarkson's Farm*, viewers get to see a tender side to Jeremy Clarkson as he worries about lambs that have been rejected by their mothers and — after years in the car industry — suddenly takes an interest in climate change. In the final episode of the first season, he calls that first year on the farm the happiest time of his life. So it is far from unusual to take a while to figure out your 'why'. Nor is that a problem. My psychology study gave me a lot of wise lessons for life, and my academic career took me to places I would never have visited otherwise. I met Nobel Prize winners, but also hundreds of victims of sexual violence and even paedophiles. I would never have had that grounding if I had chosen interior design straight away.

Even so, it is worthwhile considering your 'why' when you start a reset, says the marketing guru Simon Sinek. "Once you understand your 'why', you can specify clearly what makes you feel satisfied and you will have a better understanding of what drives you when you are at your best. If you can do that, you will have a reference point for everything you do in the future. You will be able to make more deliberate choices for your company, your career and your life. You can inspire others to buy from you, collaborate with you and share your opinions. You must never again act based on decisions taken for reasons you don't really understand. From now on, you can be goal-driven. From now on, you can start with your 'why'."

Sinek uses the image of the Golden Circle. The outer ring represents what you do, the middle ring how you do it and the inner circle why you do it. According to Sinek, the inner circle should be your point of departure in your actions and your communication. Sinek sees the Golden Circle first and foremost as a marketing strategy. A well-known example that he refers to regularly is Apple's marketing. In its communications, Apple emphasizes its vision rather than the technical specifications of its products. Why did they develop this new product? Why do you need the latest iPhone or iWatch? And that works. The same applies to you. If you actively search for your 'why' and then act accordingly — for example, by going to work for an organization that addresses your 'why' — you will feel energized. After all, you will be doing a job you love rather than just working to pay the rent. You will also find you talk more enthusiastically about your work as a result, and that will help you inspire others to come and work for you, partner with you or become your customer.

BE TRUE TO YOURSELF

Glennon Doyle's daughter said to her one evening at bedtime, "I'm big, Mum. I'm bigger than the other girls. Why am I different?" The American self-help guru was not surprised. "My daughter and I pay attention. We know what the world wants from us. We know we must decide whether to stay small, quiet, and uncomplicated or allow ourselves to grow as big, loud, and complex as we were made to be. Every girl must decide whether to be true to herself or true to the world. Every girl must decide whether to settle for adoration or fight for love." Doyle decided to be true to herself but only after she had overcome bulimia and alcoholism. Since then, she has been inspiring her followers on social media with her ground-breaking honesty. In her third book, *Untamed*, she shows women how to be themselves and liberate themselves from the expectations the world imposes on them. I find the questions she raises fascinating. Who were we before the world taught us who we should be? What do we genuinely do of our own free will and what is learned behaviour?

If you have read my previous books, you will know that I too have been on a journey over the past few years to become truer to my authentic self. Each book was a personal quest. I started with a story about how I could gain more control over my own life and avoid a bore-out. In *Het Nieuwe Mentaal*, I talked about needing courage to take radical decisions and create a new mindset. And since my third book *AI*, about authentic intelligence and the uniqueness of the human brain, I have led a more authentic life. I worry much less about what other people think. Instead, I strive for deeper connections. Like Doyle, I am prepared to let go of everyone for whom I have to keep part of myself hidden. "I shook off that fear," she said to the Dutch newspaper *Het Parool*, "and that removed three quarters of the anxiety in my life." I can relate to that. In the past, I would never have been so open about my relationship problems, but now I am prepared to share them — albeit with some trepidation — with the readers of this book. It feels incredibly liberating not to have to hide those thoughts. I am also more inclined to give my imagination free rein and to form my own opinions, regardless of what is considered chic and politic. That authenticity in my life has led me to make choices that are much more in keeping with my true self.

NEVER, EVER COPY-PASTE

My children spend their weekends with my ex and the weekdays with me. A lot of people find that a strange setup. My former partner has more quality time while I get the hassle of the school run and swimming lessons. But I chose it deliberately because I think that of the two of us, I am the more nurturing. I could also have gone for the more standard 'alternate weeks' arrangement. Then I too would have had some weekends, but I might also have started to worry about the girls missing their swimming lessons during the weeks they spent with their father, and so forth.

What is more, this basic arrangement was the starting point for my ideas about how I wanted to craft my life after my divorce. I engaged a nanny who could take the children to school and get them meals, and I made sure I could work flexible hours. But the longer the lockdown continued, the less use there seemed to be for a nanny. I was working from home anyway so I could easily take the children to school. Anyway, I didn't want to lose out on potential quality time during the week now that I was not seeing my children at the weekends. So I decided quite soon to do the tasks myself that I had originally outsourced to the nanny, and I fully appreciated the time I gained by working from home.

At present, I am busy crafting my post-Covid life. Now that hybrid working has taken off, I don't think it will be so easy to get all staff physically in one place for a workshop. Webinars are here to stay, provided they make more of an impact than live sessions. It needs to be a fulfilling experience for both parties. So you will need a film studio if you want to stand out in this respect. At the same time, I see no need for me to go to a studio if the audience are all looking at their laptops. That is why I had a film studio installed in my house where I could continue to give my webinars. I hoped this would free up time for the things that address my 'why': my children, writing books and so on.

What I want to show with these personal examples is that I don't copy-paste. *Never, ever.* I didn't copy the divorce arrangements my friends made because they didn't fit the characters of my ex and myself. I didn't copy the pre-Covid school run when I suddenly found myself spending more time at home. And when I work from home, that is not a copy of what I do when I work at the office. At the office, my desire for human contact may be satisfied by a chat with someone I bump into on the stairs. I don't bump into anyone at home but I don't get distracted either. So after having concentrated hard on my work for a few hours, I will sometimes meet up with a friend for coffee at two in the afternoon.

Deliberately crafting your life sounds easy but that is not always the case in practice. You are continually plagued by internal and external voices trying to persuade you to take a different approach (i.e. the same one as everyone else). For example, when I visit a cafe at the weekend, all I see is families with children, making me miss my daughters intensely. Or a CEO will ask me whether I could come to the firm's office after all to give my talk. The chimpanzee in me – my supposedly primitive brain – with the urge to say 'yes' to everyone, is tempted to please the CEO by consenting immediately to their request. Saying 'no' to these internal and external voices is a lot harder, even when you know deep down inside that what they want is not right for you. After all, we are conditioned to say 'yes' to questions. So how do I manage to exit the 'yes' highway? By asking a counter-question, for example "Why would I do that?" That buys me some time for reflection and puts me in greater control of my impulses.

Another crucial aspect is to draw up a schedule. "If you fail to plan, you plan to fail." If you don't schedule your new habits, they will remain vague intentions that you can easily brush aside every time you get a request. That does not mean you can't revise your schedule. A reset is not a one-off action; it is a process of continually improving and evaluating.

ROUTINES PROVIDE STABILITY (PLUS A DISCLAIMER)

"Decisions — sometimes they drive me mad.

What are we going to eat?

What should I wear, because it's hot indoors and raining outside? What on Earth are the kids going to do today?

My poor brain can't always cope, so the fewer decisions I have to take, the better.

One of my ninja tricks is if possible to take a decision that eliminates a hundred others. That's a trick I once learned from Tim Ferriss.

Years ago, I decided that I would always give personalized baby presents as the parents always think their brand-new baby's name is amazing. So I have always done the same thing since then: a name on something that fits with the parents. It has saved me hours trying to work out whether to go for a cake or a voucher.

I decided I wouldn't do Twitter. I decided I would never finish a book I wasn't enjoying after the first hundred pages. I decided I wouldn't eat before lunch. That I wouldn't wear or buy high heels. That I would only drink sparkling water and coffee. That I wouldn't do commercial partnerships and would never buy anything over the phone. All these decisions mean I never have to think about this again. Sometimes there is an advantage to restricting your thoughts and doubts.

In 2016, I decided once and for all that I would never drink alcohol again, after years of weighing up the pros and cons on every occasion.

Should I? Shouldn't I? Lots? Just a drop? Water in between? After six? It was so exhausting.

On holiday, we visited the impressive cellars of the champagne house Moët et Chandon. I thought the place was amazing, and afterwards it was simple: I didn't drink any because I don't drink. Even better: I don't have doubts either.

Not even when Youri did drink some. Because you know, I've drunk more than enough champagne in my day to know what it tastes like. I'm good."

This was what blogger Kelly Deriemaeker wrote on social media after a trip to the Champagne region. As she says, crafting your own life is fascinating but it is also incredibly tiring. Making decisions costs time and energy. Another person besides Kelly who understood this was Steve Jobs. He wore exactly the same suit every day so that he could save his energy for his creative priorities. I personally wouldn't choose to wear the same clothes every day as I get a positive vibe from selecting a stylish outfit and don't mind trying a few combinations until I have got the right one. But I can understand why this worked for Steve Jobs. Fashion didn't address his 'why'. By wearing this uniform, he freed up space in his brain for technological innovations.

The advantage of a routine or ritual like this is that it not only saves you energy, it gives you a sense of control and security. Whether you choose to end your day with a cup of tea and your diary, or not to check your smartphone until you have drawn the curtains, a routine is a kind of anchor giving you stability, and an antidote to anxiety in turbulent times. That is precisely why so many elite sportspeople are attached to their rituals. Real Madrid goalkeeper Thibaut Courtois, for example, always sends a text to his girlfriend before a match telling her he is about to get changed. Then he takes his shoes and socks off, first the left one then the right, and the same applies to the gloves. When he gets to the goal, first he taps the left post, then the right post and finally the crossbar. These rituals let him start the match with self-confidence.

Routines not only make you feel you are in control but they always help you remember things. Going swimming every Monday morning is easier than finding a time to go when you are in the mood for a swim. For example, I do a seven-minute workout every morning, so I can start the day fully energized.

Yet I have to admit that that workout is one of the few routines in my life. Even a daily task like preparing packed lunches is not a fixed ritual for me. One time I might do it the evening before, the next time in the morning before breakfast and there are also occasions when I have yet to decide what goes in the lunchbox five minutes before we are due to leave. I find it difficult to relate to the examples I gave above, even though I know in theory that they would make my life a lot easier.

For a long time I did not know why I have such an aversion to routine, until I realized that my dislike of fixed rituals was directly related to my focus on growth. I am afraid I would stagnate if I were to pack the lunchboxes at exactly the same time every day, following a fixed weekly menu. That may be a little excessive: there are plenty of areas where I could continue to grow even with such a packed lunch routine. Still...

That is why this particular life-crafting guideline comes with a warning: incorporate routines in your life, but break them every now and again. Check that you can still function without that routine, that you can cope if you do things differently for one day. Certainly in post-COVID-19 times, you need to be alert to this because as philosopher Ignaas Devisch wrote in an essay in August 2021, "Anyone who restricts their lives to the familiar or the routine is at risk of ending up in a kind of existential obsessional neurosis. The pandemic has reinforced this neurosis. It restricted our mobility and forced our relations with other people into a straitjacket. Have any of us got to know new people in the past eighteen months? [...] Of course we need to plan and organize things a little but our lives would be a great deal poorer if we were to limit this reboot of our social lives to the planned-efficient dimension and dispense with the explorative-adventurous dimension of our existence. Life is the result not just of what you deliberately aim for but also what happens to you and cannot be grasped so firmly."

TAKE YOUR TIME... NOT

"Take all the time you need." How often have you heard these words after a setback? I too have regularly been given that well-meant advice. But you will never hear me say this: not if an employee announces a divorce, not if a friend is sacked from her job and not if a CEO's company has recorded a loss. That doesn't mean I don't try to be empathic but why should I advise someone facing a reversal of fortune to mope around? Where does that get them?

In my opinion, the employee doesn't first need to process his divorce before taking on a new challenge at work, or deciding to sign up for the New York marathon or even before starting a new romantic relationship. A new track can actually help you to process the setback. There is no need whatsoever for a long standstill. I too have been prepared to keep going during difficult periods. Indeed, you will never find me mentioning the word 'regret'. You only waste valuable time and energy if you mope about your problems.

Yet I regularly see people wallowing in their victimhood. For example, one of my clients was in a tricky situation a few years ago. Her life was in a mess because her daughter had left the family home at the age of 20 after a conflict and moved in with her boyfriend. My client blamed "that boy" for the rift between mother and daughter and denied she personally had any share in what had happened. One year later, she was still not ready to move on. She fixated on the past and idealized it. So she ended up in a bubble where she was the victim. She was unable to take a step back and reflect on what had happened and how she could get on with her life.

Not long ago she learned that her daughter was pregnant. I saw that might be an opening for her to get out of her rut, so I invited her to a Zoom session. I confronted her with the fact that she only has one life; she'd only become a grandmother for the first time once. Even if things had been said that still hurt her, that was no reason not to focus on her new role as grandmother or not to support her daughter during this unique period. Moving on is the only way to grow. Or as the poet Yung Pueblo put it so aptly: "Throw away the idea that you need to pause your life until you are fully healed, this is a different way of being attached to perfection. Progress happens when you make better decisions in the midst of living."

FLIP-THINKING

"My work diary is empty. All my lectures have been cancelled," I sighed on the phone to a friend at the start of the pandemic. "But I haven't got time to chat on the phone," I added. "I'm rushing from one meeting to the next." "Hang on," said my friend. "Don't put the phone down yet. I don't get it. Your diary is empty and yet you're complaining you don't have enough time — not for me, not for your daughters. That can't be right." "Sorry, I really haven't got time," I said quickly. My third video meeting of the morning was about to start. It was only in the break between the fourth and fifth video calls of the day that I found a few minutes to reflect on her words. I could really do with more time for myself, and with the divorce I felt my daughters needed that time too. Why did I carry on working so hard when my schedule was literally empty? Of course, crisis plans had to be made but at that point in the pandemic, I didn't need to be doing that from first thing in the morning to last thing at night. We had come up with a plan and we suspected that once the crisis had abated, the demand from companies for support for mental welfare would be greater than ever. So it would work out all right in the end. Perhaps I should no longer see the empty work diary as an insurmountable problem but rather as a welcome break, an opportunity to reconnect with myself and gather my strength. From that time on, I grouped my work meetings in the mornings, the afternoons were for my daughters and after they had been put to bed, I did the activities that gave me energy. I believe it was on one such evening that I got the idea for this book.

By inverting my thinking about the situation, I stopped just seeing the obstacles in the situation and was able to see the opportunities as well. When I look back now, it seems incredibly obvious. Once you have flipped a thought, you can't imagine not thinking that way, but at the time I was stuck in the old thought pattern for several weeks.

Flip-thinking is a concept proposed by Berthold Gunster. It is a technique for reframing your problems and transforming them into possibilities. Flip-thinking is the opposite of inflexible thinking — where your thoughts are stuck in a rut — a typical thought pattern in which the problems only get bigger. Inflexible thinkers say "yes, but..." whenever someone offers them a solution, and they focus exclusively on the obstacles associated with this possible route to success. Gunster argues that flip-thinking is superior to inflexible thinking but also to solving: "You want to get more out of a problem, because it leads you directly to a new opportunity." That certainly applies to me. The emptier my work diary became, the more room there was in my brain to work out the concept for this book. The more free afternoons I had, the better I was able to support my daughters in what was such an emotional time for them. It goes without saying that they enjoyed having me around. We had more quality time than ever before. When my diary started to fill up again a few months later and the free afternoons became increasingly rare, I feared they would be disappointed. But when I told the girls — with some hesitation — that my work was starting to get busier again, to my surprise they broke into smiles. "That means we can go to Granny and Grandad's more often again," they said, beaming. I clearly didn't need to teach my daughters the art of flip-thinking.

WHAT IF YOU FLY?

A reset is no walk in the park or an American-style dream come true. There are downsides too. "It is a mistake to want everything to be 'fun, fun, fun'" is one of psychiatrist Dirk De Wachter's pet subjects. In my book *Het Nieuwe Mentaal*, I wrote about "daring to choose to be out of balance". You need to learn to accept that risks are part of life. If you can't do that, you will always be afraid and that anxiety will keep you at a standstill. I could have thought to myself "What if my relationship with Bert doesn't work out?" Then I would never have dared take the step of buying a house together.

Really, there is only one appropriate answer to that question: "What would I do if it didn't work out?" The biggest mistake people make is believing that your life ends when you have one failure. They can't imagine that life can still go on even after a crisis or failure. Unconvinced? Check how someone is doing a couple of years after a drama. Look up that family who lost their house in a fire, the young father who had to manage alone after his wife died, the teenager who ended up in a coma after a traffic accident. Their lives didn't end after that drama — on the contrary. As a business owner, I have been fascinated by the Fuckup Nights movement, network events in which entrepreneurs share stories of their failures. The aim is to break the taboo of failure and focus on the lessons that can be learned from the experience. That we have some way to go is illustrated by the comments of the former judoka Heidi Rakels, one of the leading lights of the Failing Forward campaign: "If you make a mistake in Europe, you soon get a stigma. If you just miss bronze in Sydney, you're labelled a loser. Whereas in the US they say, 'Fantastic! You took part in the Olympics!'" Just as elite athletes lose more often than they win, Rakels was not afraid to start her own company, "because you only really lose when you don't even try".

Like Heidi with her company, I made myself vulnerable by daring to go for a new relationship and not allowing myself to be immobilized by "What if it doesn't work out?" If it fails, that will cause me a lot of pain. But isn't vulnerability at the root of all the wonderful things in life? Or as the professor and expert in shame and vulnerability Brené Brown says, "Vulnerability is the birthplace of innovation, creativity and change." I decided that if there was a possibility that this step would make me happier, I should seize the opportunity. And perhaps there is a second answer to the question "What if it doesn't work out?" *Oh but my darling, what if you fly?*

After I told my network that my husband and I were separating, I received two e-mails that same day. Colleagues wrote that they had wanted to leave their partner for years but didn't know how to manage it. Even though their children were much older than mine, they didn't dare take control and reset their lives. Precisely because they had invested so many years in the relationship, a reset felt like they were giving up. They had the notion that they had chosen a particular path and now they had to stick to it. They had ended up in a steady state of languishing. They didn't have the reflex that you can always transform your life at any time.

A status quo bias in which you have a preference for the as-is situation is a known phenomenon in psychology. We prefer to play safe rather than try something new. But why do we do that? Why do managers often find it so difficult to get their team on board when the company is restructured? Why do you often find yourself saying "That's how we do things here" when your kids ask why different rules apply at their friend's house? And why does your partner still make spaghetti sauce according to their mother's recipe? The answer is simple: making a change requires an effort and the outcome is uncertain.

People who lack confidence in a positive outcome often do not have the self-discipline to change direction. "Because I've already put in so much effort," they often say. "I've spent so many years studying for this profession, invested so much in this house, taken so much time to perfect this recipe that it would be a shame to throw that all away." We call this 'effort justification': we attach more value to something that we put a lot of effort into than things that cost us no effort. This notion underlies Ikea's whole philosophy. We appreciate a bookcase we put together ourselves more than one where we didn't have to spend hours following instructions. It sounds logical but there is a risk associated with effort justification. The emotions evoked by the effort invested prevent you from seeing clearly and making rational decisions.

In fact, changing our opinions and altering course from time to time is crucial to our mental wellbeing, as you can only grow then. And it is never too late, even after you have spent years investing in another direction. Let's put an end to the notion that we can never start at a new company in a junior position after the age of 40 or that we can never take up a new hobby. There are plenty of inspiring examples of the fallacy of this idea. Journalist and figure skater Vera Wang started in the fashion business when she was 40 and now looks just as good in her seventies as women half her age. Actor Ronald Reagan peaked even later, only standing for governor at the age of 54, yet he went on to become the president of the United States. And most elite sportspeople have to make a switch half-way through their working lives.

LOVINGLY STRICT

The concept of self-compassion comes from Kristin Neff, an American psychology professor. She discovered that self-compassion is the counterpart of self-criticism and shame, two bugbears of mental health. Countless studies show that if you make progress with a psychologist, self-criticism and shame can completely undo all that progression. Self-compassion, on the other hand, means that rather than constantly criticizing yourself, you treat yourself as you would a good friend. You wouldn't tell a friend who failed at something "How could you be so stupid?" whereas our carping inner voice is quite capable of saying something like that.

A little self-compassion is necessary if you want a reset because every reset inevitably involves some failures. Yet we tend to associate this concept with complacency and taking it easy. As an advocate of more ownership and willpower, I too used to be rather sceptical about the idea. But self-compassion expert Elke Smeets has taught me that self-compassion does not have to be a synonym for spoiling yourself. "Self-compassion doesn't mean that you always have to pamper yourself; you can also be lovingly strict. For example, you might say to yourself, 'OK, you're tired but you should still go to the gym. You'll probably feel better afterwards'. But not 'It would be really bad if you skipped gym class yet again. You'll get fatter and fatter, you lazy fool!' Self-compassion is about creating self-care instead of self-harm."

A GOAL THAT IS GREATER THAN YOURSELF

"Would someone go to the recycling centre for me if I paid them? Some large items need to be taken there and I don't have a trailer," I typed somewhat hesitantly in Hoplr, an app that brings neighbours in contact with one another. I got a response just two hours later. A retired couple — Josée and Mark — could drop by the next afternoon and take everything. "I'll pay you," I promised them the next day when they arrived at my door. "There's really no need; we've got the time," Josée assured me.

It was the first time I had asked for help via the app. I had previously offered help myself by giving away baby clothes and keeping seniors in the neighbourhood company. Of course I could have hired a trailer or van this time or called the second-hand shop for them to collect the items we no longer wanted, but that would have been a transaction and not worth mentioning in this book. Thanks to Josée and Mark, it became an act of solidarity and benevolence that immediately made me feel better: the world was full of good people. Using an app also made it a very hybrid deed. Technology *can* bring people together, and I would never have found this couple without Hoplr.

Of course I couldn't help asking my generous village neighbours why they were prepared to sacrifice a free afternoon to take stuff to the recycling centre for a complete stranger. Wouldn't they rather do something fun and enjoy their retirement? "We like to make ourselves useful," was their reply. "Sure it's nice to sit outside at a pub or go on a day trip, and we'll probably be doing that tomorrow. But that pint will taste even better if we can look back with satisfaction at what we did for you today."

What Josée and Mark have discovered is that happiness has multiple levels. Many people confuse happiness with a pleasurable life: spoiling yourself when you go shopping, eating out at top restaurants and so on. That is all very well but a pleasurable life soon becomes hedonistic and can eventually seem 'empty'.

The next level of happiness is the flow state you get into when you are doing something you love and are good at. You lose track of time and are almost on a high. This level is closely related to resilience. The American professor of psychology Martin Seligman has also identified a third level of happiness, that of the meaningful life. At this level, you use your strengths to contribute to a goal that is greater than yourself. That gives you a much deeper sense of satisfaction than an evening out at a pub with your friends.

KEEP IT SIMPLE

One of my favourite thinkers — who I have already mentioned a couple of times in this book — is Yuval Noah Harari. I draw inspiration from how he can sum up our complex world in a few sentences with his macro-analyses. Harari does not get bogged down in unnecessary details; he filters messy reality to extract the essence. There is huge power in that simplicity. In complex times, we long for an overview.

While my life may look complicated to an outsider, with my

reconfigured family and my own company, I actually like to keep things simple. Yes, really! Nobody is more likely than me to ask themselves, "Should I be doing this now?" The technique I use is to repeat the question multiple times, stressing a different word in the sentence each time. *Should* I be cooking an Instagram-worthy meal now or have I just talked myself into it? Should *I* be laying out the children's clothes now for the next morning or could they choose their own outfits? Should I be answering that e-mail *now* or could I run through all my e-mails at the same time later? Should I be *cycling at top speed for an hour* now or would a recreational cycle trip also do? Should I be *doing* that job or is it unnecessary? Asking this question lets me eliminate at least half the must-dos in my life.

Furthermore, I can accept that life is sometimes complex. If all the kids are at home, I don't have a minute-by-minute plan for the day; I just let it all happen. I am open to the surprises that a day with four children brings. Instead of trying to work my way through an enormous to-do list, I make sure we do something that gives us energy. But my principal simplifying strategy is to live in the here-and-now. If I have a Saturday without the kids, I don't run through the scenario of the past week or coming week in my head. If I'm on holiday with my partner, I don't have my mind on the preparations for the next team meeting. And if I'm giving a talk, I don't start thinking about the new design for our garden. That seems obvious, but in practice it is anything but.

WE NEED PEOPLE TO RESHAPE OUR WORLD

"Humanity as a whole has so far failed to contain the pandemic, or to devise a global plan to defeat the virus. The early months of 2020 were like watching an accident in slow motion. Modern communication made it possible for people all over the world to see in real time the images first from Wuhan, then from Italy, then from more and more countries – but no global leadership emerged to stop the catastrophe from engulfing the world." I am quoting Yuval Noah Harari once again.

What Harari describes is a reactive policy that started on the back foot. Where were the brave politicians with a global action plan at the start of the crisis? Where was the plan that not only aimed at containing the pandemic but also took into account other interests and values? And thinking of global welfare, where were the policymakers one year later when the first vaccines could have been shared equally? Where are the politicians who can shape our post-Covid world?

We need people to reshape our world. This is where policymakers can make the difference. If it is just a question of interpreting curves, a computer can tell you which measures are most effective. Computers are better able to determine what should be done to contain the pandemic than any individual human. However, authentic and intelligent policymakers look at the bigger picture. They are prepared to take a step back and with every decision they take, ask "Is this beneficial for humanity as a whole?" They are willing to choose change.

Time for a reset

"But when are you going to get onto the topic of work?" asked my publisher somewhat anxiously when I sent her the first half of my manuscript. "With Better Minds at Work, you are mainly known as a wellbeing expert for companies but the first 100 pages of your book is about us as individuals. I thought this was going to be a book about hybrid work?"

"The individual is the determining factor in the success of hybrid work," I explained. "You can only introduce this new way of working once employees have sufficient resilience, understand how their brain functions in a crisis and know about the tools to start a reset. Otherwise you risk provoking resistance. And you don't want that, because hybrid work has huge potential."

"OK, but when are you going to get onto the topic of work?" she repeated. (My publisher is not one to give up easily.)

"Now," I told her.

CHAPTER 4

THE BRAIN IS KEY IN THE NEW WAY OF WORKING

WHY HYBRID WORK IS HERE TO STAY

The best of both worlds

Lisa, the head of HR at a large company, is chairing a selection panel. She finalizes the details for a new recruitment action with her management team. She has done one online interview after another over the past few weeks, discussing matters with her colleagues in between in Teams meetings. She hardly has time during the day to record her findings and reply to her e-mails, so she does that in the evenings, after the children have gone to bed.

Lisa works in her bedroom. To give a more professional impression, she has selected a blurred background. She has hung up a large wall planner on the door to her bedroom so that her children can see when they come home from school when Mum is at work.

The selection panel has finished, Lisa clicks the 'leave Teams' button — and bursts into tears. The many months of working from home without her colleagues but with a full diary have taken their toll. Not to mention the tough weeks when the schools were closed and she had to become a teacher on top of her full-time job in HR. Her energy and willpower are depleted, her mental resilience damaged. She can't wait to get back to the office.

A GLOBAL EXPERIMENT IN RESILIENCE

During the health crisis in 2020 and 2021, we all experienced similar or even greater mental challenges at work and ran up against our own point of no return. In fact, you can clearly conclude that the crisis was a global experiment in resilience at work. And still is, because the experiment is continuing.

At the start of the pandemic, millions of people suddenly had to work from home, creating improvised desks or clearing the kitchen table in their houses or flats, and juggling online meeting schedules. Our rigidly structured and optimized lives — our pre-pandemic lives that we had packed full with work appointments, training courses, hobbies, trips and social and family engagements — came to a standstill at the start of the crisis, and our diaries were wiped clean.

I too saw one appointment after another cancelled in the spring of 2020. It was quite a shock. My working life changed dramatically, from interactive talks with a live audience and exchanging ideas with colleagues at the office to webinars and online meetings. I recorded the webinars in our empty office to get myself into work mode, as it were. It felt weird standing in front of the camera all alone. Even now, I still feel a shiver go down my spine when I enter our office building and am reminded of the challenges of the first lockdown.

Initially, we rolled up our sleeves and enthusiastically made the best of it. We weren't going to let this exceptional situation get the better of us. We would prove how flexible we could be. Hey, now we actually had more productive hours. We no longer wasted time on the daily commute, coffee breaks with colleagues or pointless meetings. Most employers and employees were in attack mode in March 2020, when the first lockdown was introduced. Together, we would sort this problem out.

We also gradually discovered that there were benefits to working from home. Less time spent in traffic freed up a lot of hours for us. Young parents no longer had those stress peaks in the mornings and evenings, and experienced unexpected quality moments with their kids. Some employees found that they could clear the mind by exercising or going on a walk during the working day, and that this let them concentrate better, perform their tasks more efficiently and perhaps even get in an undisturbed flow. I also found that family life became less stressed because I was able to take my children to school and pick them up again in the afternoon. I more than made up for those 'lost' working hours in the evenings.

THE SAME BUT DIFFERENT

Even so, not everyone was so defiant and upbeat, or able to keep that up in the longer term. Suspicious companies that had never been that keen on working from home felt they were now saddled with a problem. They wondered whether their staff would be as productive at home as they were at the office. Some managers and HR departments went into overdrive, installing spyware on their employees' PCs to monitor their productivity and attention span or even their online surfing — forgetting that by doing this, they were damaging their employees' oh-so-valuable trust for good. Employees who feel their boss is constantly checking up on them and restricting them in their work are less productive. In the long term, they are more likely to undermine the company's objectives than support them. You could dub this approach Operation Mistrust.

But even the managers and employees who initially embraced remote work realized after the first few weeks of the pandemic that there are fundamental differences between working at an office and working from home. It is not a question of copy-paste.

Working from home demands a tailored approach, and that approach does not consist of filling the working day with back-to-back digital appointments or organizing large meetings with thirty heads on the screen on mute. Add the need to continually reply to e-mails and WhatsApp messages and you have the recipe for an inefficient, unfocused day spent working from home.

THE START OF HYBRID WORK

When the measures were relaxed bit by bit, we saw the start of a hybrid approach to work. Just as we had finally got used to working from home all the time, we had to make a new change. Some people were desperate to get back to the office (if only part of the time) while others had become attached to working from home and preferred to keep it that way.

But whether you are an office fan or a homebody, you will undoubtedly have found out first hand that constantly switching between home and the office brings its own challenges. It is not just the fact that you always need to have the right files with you but also the fact that your team will often no longer all be in the same place at the same time. If you always work at the office, it is easy to arrange a meeting. The same goes if you are all working from home. But what if five of you are in an open-plan office but you still have to have a video conference because three other employees work from home on that day?

In my conversations with managers, I see that they are not always positive in their evaluations of the first experiments with hybrid work. "It is a real hassle coordinating everyone's diaries" or "I get the impression the team members are working alongside but not *with* one another." So they hope they will soon be able to return to the old normal. "We may keep one day working from home, but in general I would prefer staff to all be working together at the office."

What a missed opportunity. I admit that just as we all had to learn how to work from home when the coronavirus crisis started, so it may take a while before we have mastered hybrid work. But I am absolutely convinced that hybrid work is the future, precisely because it has huge potential in letting us find a way of working that is aligned with what our brains need. Fortunately other points of view are being heard too. Gartner estimates that almost two thirds of employees — mainly knowledge workers — will be able to work remotely at least some of the time.

Companies that opt for a hybrid model are taking various routes. Some are choosing a more flexible approach. At IBM, for example, the number of days an employee works in the office depends on their tasks and whether they need to collaborate in teams. Office workers at Ford need to come to the office for certain meetings or projects but can work from home on individual tasks. Other companies such as Uber, Swift and Citigroup require staff to come to the office a certain number of days a week, usually two or three days. At the other end of the spectrum, some employers are dividing employees into categories or tiers. The company Salesforce has three categories: flex (one to three days a week at the office), remote full-time and at the office full-time (four to five days a week).

Whatever hybrid scheme companies come up with, it is striking that their decisions are largely based on practical arguments. Of course it is useful to make a financial cost-benefit analysis. If you expand working from home and decrease office space, this can undoubtedly lead to savings in the longer term. But if you only consider this aspect of the issue, you may miss the many other benefits from choosing the right approach to work — benefits for both the individual employees and the company as a whole. Greater productivity, more efficiency, better and more creative work, happier workers — surely all these factors should be taken into account too?

Microsoft CEO Satya Nadella describes the situation as follows: "In the past year, no domain has undergone a more rapid transformation than how we work. Employees' expectations are changing and we will need to define productivity more broadly — to include collaboration, learning and welfare with the aim of boosting the career development of all employees, including front-line staff and knowledge workers, as well as recent graduates and those who currently make up the professional classes. This should all be done with flexibility in when, where and how people work."

I hope this book will serve as an invitation to the stakeholders — companies, employees and society as a whole — to reflect on how we can incorporate the many positive experiences of working from home in a new post-Covid regime for work. Hybrid work is here to stay. The tipping point has been reached. It is up to us to get the most out of this reset.

THE BIGGEST MISCONCEPTION ABOUT HYBRID WORK IS...

Hybrid work is not the implementation of specific agreements about time and place, nor is it a transition. Hybrid work is a transformation of how we all do our work. It affects the essence of our 'labour'. Or as HR specialist Josh Bersin puts it, "We are not 'going back' to the office, we are 'going forward' to a new, hybrid work culture."

THE FOUR DIMENSIONS OF PRODUCTIVITY

What makes an employee productive? In most jobs, there are four dimensions to productivity in addition to time (working at the right moment) and place (working in a location that is adapted to the type of work you need to do). These four dimensions are energy, focus, coordination and collaboration. A job gives you a certain degree of personal energy and focus, but there are times when you need to coordinate matters with colleagues or clients, or collaborate with co-workers, other departments or external partners on projects. Each of these four dimensions can have a positive or negative impact on productivity.

Energy

A job can recharge your batteries, energize you and increase your vitality, but it can also sap your energy and lead to fatigue and apathy.

Focus

If you are focused, you can concentrate fully and get in a flow state where time flies by. It's that wonderful feeling where you lose track of time and suddenly think "Oh, is it that late?!" after having got a huge amount of work done. That is when you are at your most productive. But sometimes even minor distractions are enough to make you lose concentration, or you feel obliged to flit constantly between projects, multi-tasking and never getting any satisfaction from the work you deliver.

Coordination

If the coordination with your team members or clients goes smoothly, you can work efficiently and effectively. You can feel that you'll get results. But if there are any hitches in the coordination for whatever reason, it can be counterproductive and you risk mistakes being made.

Collaboration

Collaborating on a particular project can give you a good vibe and lead to better results if there is room for cooperation and participation, if you are safely and constructively valued as an employee and if you can make use of your talents. But if there are internal or external disruptive elements, the collaboration can soon lead to resistance and competition between people.

As employees, we function best when we can combine flexibility in time and place with these four dimensions of productivity *and* if we can check them against the brain criterion.

THE BRAIN CRITERION

Even since I founded Better Minds at Work, I have been stressing how important it is to understand how our brains work and above all to make decisions based on that knowledge. Ideally, any changes we make to our way of working should take the brain as the starting point. With every reset, we should ask ourselves, "Is this brain-friendly?"

Let me give a simple example. Many companies plan team meetings first thing in the morning, at nine o'clock. That is when our brains are at their most alert, time that would therefore be better used for deep work. Meetings at the start of the working day are wasted brain time and consequently harm productivity. They require much less focus than writing a report, coordinating a project or coming up with a strategy, so you are better off planning them at times when we generally find it harder to get in a mental flow, for example just after lunch. That way, you keep the alert-brain mornings free for the tasks that require the most concentration.

OF ELEPHANTS AND RABBITS

I discussed the metaphor of the elephants and the rabbits in my book *Mentaal kapitaal*. The basis for this was a quote from the Texan oil magnate and billionaire Thomas Boone Pickens: “When you are hunting elephants, don’t get distracted chasing rabbits.” The elephants represent the priorities on the horizon, and you will usually adopt a strategy to hunt them. The rabbits in the meantime are jumping all over the place, and you want to hunt them down as quickly as possible.

To divide up your working day or working week optimally, you need to determine your priorities and more minor tasks in advance. Then tackle them in that order: first the elephants, then the rabbits. Having a clearly defined objective (the elephants) is one of the key prerequisites for getting in a flow. You can reward yourself afterwards with the rabbits, such as e-mails and phone calls. This technique lets you tackle the important tasks when your body and mind have most energy – usually in the morning.

Elephant time can also be scheduled by a company. For example, a manager at a leading international construction company scheduled ‘elephant time’ for her entire department on my recommendation. Staff work undisturbed on their projects every day between nine and eleven; meetings are never scheduled during this period. They are not distracted by the ‘rabbits’, the more minor assignments that require less focus.

A manager at an insurance company asked for our help after he noted that staff in the customer service centre were unable to focus. They spent the whole day switching between the demanding cases (the elephants) and the phone ringing with new claims (the rabbits). This way of working was not very productive. Together, we were able to find a solution. Now, half the employees concentrate on the cases for two hours while the other half deal with the phone calls. After two hours, they swap round. The staff experience a better balance between intensive and light work, the cases are dealt with better – because staff can focus more – and new customers don't get stressed employees on the other end of the line. It is a win-win situation.

See the clip about elephants and rabbits
on the Mental Reset video channel.

Making hybrid happen!

SYNCHRONOUS VERSUS ASYNCHRONOUS

First things first. What exactly do we mean by hybrid work? We almost automatically think of flexibility in time and place.

As regards 'place', we traditionally think of the home or the office. 'Home' means your house or flat, your garden, the corner coffee shop or even a holiday location abroad. Any place where you can work efficiently as an employee counts. By 'office' we mean not only a traditional workplace but also satellite offices and co-working hubs.

Flexibility in time means specifically that the working hours can vary from one employee to the next. If you are at work at the same time as the other team members, your work is synchronous. Asynchronous means that you are at work at times when other team members are not. For example, if one team member is an evening person who works best late and the others are not, the work is asynchronous. The same applies when young parents take a few hours off in the afternoon and compensate by working in the evening. But asynchronous can also mean you are at work at the same time as the others but are temporarily unavailable because you want to concentrate on a particular task without any interruption.

Any company that wants to work out a sound policy for hybrid work should therefore say goodbye to fixed days and times: no more working days from nine to five and no more working weeks from Monday to Friday.

These fixed times and the associated processes of clocking in and time recording — which are unfortunately still standard practice in some organizations — are based on an outdated view of work. Having fixed times is not good for productivity. That became clear to far more people during the pandemic. Nobody has the willpower to concentrate for eight hours without a break. The average attention span of an adult is between 30 and 45 minutes. Then you need a short break. If we want to plan our workdays in a brain-friendly way, the schedule needs to be built around our personal and collective attention curves. And why shouldn't those hours and days evolve in line with our phase of life? People in their twenties might prefer a lie-in while young parents might like to end work earlier. In a hybrid working environment, employees will be largely free to decide this for themselves.

THE FOUR DIMENSIONS OF PRODUCTIVITY IN HYBRID TIMES

If you shake off the old ideas about work and when it should be done, you gain real freedom to achieve a genuine shift that boosts the mental capital of both individual employees and the organization as a whole. If you go for hybrid work, you will be able to allow for the abovementioned four dimensions of productivity: energy, collaboration, focus and coordination. Each of these productivity dimensions flourishes best in combination with a certain place (home, office or elsewhere) and/or a certain time setup (synchronous or asynchronous). At Better Minds at Work, we used this as the basis for a handy, practical arrangement for individuals or whole teams.

Energy

Most people find it easier to restore their energy levels at home rather than at the office. Time spent working from home is productive in recharging your batteries. This is time when you can concentrate fully on the content and work efficiently without interruption and when you get a lot of satisfaction from your task. In other words, this dimension is most likely to boost productivity when combined with flexibility in the place of work.

But if you spend too much time working from home alone with only digital contact with co-workers, that can sap your energy. In such circumstances, a face-to-face meeting or sociable lunch break with the team can be a genuine source of energy.

Collaboration

Flexibility in where you work is also crucial for optimum collaboration with your colleagues or business partners. If you want to brainstorm with colleagues and make rapid progress, or if you want to be able to interpret their body language during a meeting, you are best off meeting up in person. You can all come to the office but there may well be more inspiring or practical solutions, for example a meeting combined with a walk, or two days brainstorming at a seaside resort.

Focus

If you want to be able to focus at work, the obvious solution seems to be to work on your own, away from your colleagues, for example at home or in a 'focus room' at the office. But what is often forgotten, even though it is actually more important for your focus, is the time at which you work. You will only be able to concentrate fully when your work is asynchronous. After all, if your colleagues aren't working at the same time, you won't be disturbed by incoming e-mails, phone calls or WhatsApp messages. That is precisely why I sometimes like to work for a couple of hours very early in the morning or late at night. Even if working unusual hours isn't practical or effective for you, though, you can still make agreements about when and how you put the flow of incoming messages on hold.

Coordination

Finally, coordinating with customers or colleagues works best if you can bounce ideas or potential agreements off one another quickly, and that means synchronized work. However, there are enough online tools available for allocating tasks or posting status updates on your progress that an asynchronous approach is often perfectly feasible for this.

See the clip about the four dimensions of productivity
on the Mental Reset video channel.

If you take these four dimensions into account, you can decide as an employee when and where you should work. The ideal solution will vary per person and possibly also over time. For example, a job working in a call centre will require less collaboration and coordination with co-workers than a job as an events organizer. And a professor will have a greater need for focus when writing a research article than when they are setting up a research project that involves multiple departments.

Schedule some focus time every day

Research shows that after an interruption, our brains need 25 minutes to get back into a state of deep concentration. In other words, our brains are not designed for multi-tasking. Multi-taskers are up to 40 per cent less efficient. But when we are working from home, we tend to combine different tasks. We answer our e-mails while in a meeting, finish a case with the children in the room or make an important phone call while cooking a meal. We like to think we are saving time but nothing could be further from the truth. We can be digitally in multiple places at once but we can't do the same with our thoughts. All we can do is switch between tasks. So make sure that you can give your full concentration and focus to certain tasks. As I wrote above, the way to do this is to consider what your elephants and rabbits are. Once you know what your elephant is for that day, you can schedule specific focus time for it. Disable your e-mail notifications, switch to 'not available' in Teams and put anything else that might distract you, such as your smartphone, in another room.

Dare to be unreachable sometimes

In the past, being unreachable during working hours was a definite no-no, especially when working from home. However, it is not only a prerequisite if you want to schedule sufficient focus time, it is also the only way to invest in what I call 'absent time', both as an individual and as a team.

Absent time is essential recuperation time for you or your team. If you rush through the day without stopping, for example by being permanently online or having back-to-back meetings without a break, you don't give your brain a chance to process and store the information and interpret it correctly.

At the office, we find it perfectly acceptable for someone to wander off to the coffee machine or pop in on a colleague to discuss something. Teachers often need to change classrooms for the next lesson. Sales reps spend time in the car between customer visits. You may not realize it but these are all micro-moments when both you and your brain get to be offline.

It is a mistake lots of us made when the crisis first forced us to work from home: we were on the computer working for three to four hours at a stretch, fuelled by coffee. There were no co-workers to disturb you, but also no co-workers who spontaneously dropped in to let off steam or ask how your weekend was. This meant our brains were permanently in work mode. No wonder we often felt so exhausted at the end of the working day.

Microsoft's Human Factors Lab investigated the effect of back-to-back meetings without any breaks. They asked fourteen people to attend video meetings while EEC equipment measured their brain activity. On the first day, the fourteen volunteers took part in four consecutive meetings of half an hour each. Each meeting had a different topic, from designing an office floorplan to drawing up a marketing plan. On the second day, ten-minute breaks were scheduled between the four half-hour-long meetings. During the breaks, the participants meditated using the Headspace app. The study produced one crucial conclusion, namely that there is a simple antidote to meeting-induced exhaustion: take short breaks.

Breaks between meetings allow the brain to 'reset' itself, thereby avoiding an accumulation of stress. During the breaks, the beta activity in the brainwaves — the brainwave frequencies linked to stress — declined and the participants were in a more relaxed state when they joined the next meeting. The breaks also ensured that the average level of the beta waves remained stable throughout the four meetings, without the build-up of stress.

Breaks are crucial. That is why I advocate being luxuriously unreachable sometimes. Not only because it gives you an opportunity to implement some genuine focus time (don't forget your elephants and rabbits!) but also because it's impossible to be permanently switched on. Have the courage to incorporate recuperation time during your working day when your brain has reached saturation point and you have no energy left. Go offline, take a short walk and get back to work with your batteries fully recharged. And have the courage to raise the topic of being unreachable, whether with co-workers, with your manager or as a manager yourself. Dare to break down barriers and decide how to create a flow state in your team. After all, each team and each individual employee needs their own flexibility, from being permanently synchronous to almost permanently asynchronous.

Safeguard your energy

In many companies, productivity stayed the same or even increased during the pandemic. That may seem like good news at first glance but this increase in productivity was often at the expense of exhausted workers.

According to the 2021 Work Trend Index, about one in five employees say that their employer is not interested in their work-life balance, 54 per cent feel overworked and 39 per cent exhausted. We have also seen digital exhaustion. The average number of meetings and chats has increased substantially in recent months. Figures from Microsoft in 2021 show that the time spent in Teams meetings around the world has doubled and this new level has been sustained. The average Teams meeting lasts 10 minutes longer than before the pandemic. Time spent in meetings increased 125 per cent in Australia and 67 per cent in China compared with pre-Covid figures. What is more, the average Teams user sends 45 per cent more chat messages per week, while the number of chat messages per person outside working hours has increased by 42 per cent, and is still rising.

Of course, it is hardly surprising that we have been spending more time meeting and communicating online. There was often no in-person alternative. We replaced formal and informal face-to-face discussions with digital meetings, but we forgot that the way we communicate digitally can be enormously draining. The pace of virtual work is often faster, for example. Meetings are organized hyper-efficiently, and there is no time for slouching. While we are busy leaving one meeting, the host for the following meeting is already waiting for us. The same goes for e-mails and chat messages: everything seems equally urgent. What is more, messages you receive by e-mail or an app come across very differently compared with the same message in a face-to-face encounter.

If you are working from home and get an e-mail from a colleague with a short sentence such as "Could you deal with this?" then you can interpret the request in various ways. It could be quite innocent but your brain might interpret it as a command or even an accusatory question, and you start worrying about the deeper meaning. But if that same colleague comes to your desk, smiles at you and says "Could you deal with this?", your brain only needs a fraction of a second to figure out how to interpret the request from your colleague's tone of voice and body language. When we have face-to-face conversations, our brain is given the opportunity to interpret signals such as the tone of the conversation and the body language, but that is nigh on impossible in a digital environment.

In her book *Digital Body Language,* the researcher and communication specialist Erica Dhawan tries to decode the new digital signals and codes that could replace our body language. She points out how much we communicate physically by leaning forward, making eye contact, smiling, nodding, crossing our arms or looking relaxed. We show that we are listening and that we are interested in the person we are talking to. Online communication will always be different to the offline variant but there are still rules of etiquette that can help you and your colleagues avoid 'digistress'. For example, think hard about what you are saying when drafting an e-mail and make sure you provide enough context. But also make sure you read other people's e-mails carefully and don't over-interpret them. It is also important to choose the right medium at the right time. A quick app message may be fine in some circumstances but a phone call or video call is often far more effective than a thousand e-mails, says Dhawan.

Do a digital detox

I admit that during the pandemic, I too was sometimes guilty of an excess of online meetings. My diary filled up with appointments with clients. Because I know that the cognitive burden of an online meeting is much greater than for an in-person meeting, I went back to old-school phone calls for one-on-one appointments. At first, some of my clients were sceptical when I rejected the option of a video call. It felt like they were being brushed off. Wasn't their issue worth a video meeting? But their scepticism evaporated once I had them on the phone. Now that I am no longer video-calling, I have more focus and energy and I can give my clients my full, undivided attention. I was not the only one to take this approach. *Rector magnificus* of Maastricht University Rianne Letschert tweeted on 7 June 2021 "I got rid of all my Zoom appointments up to ten o'clock and made ordinary phone calls instead. Then I could go for a nice walk! You need to look after yourself sometimes. Have a good weekend, everybody."

In this regard, I can highly recommend the work of digital coach Florence Pérès, who created the Digital Balance Programme at Better Minds at Work. In her book *Digital Detox,* she explains why our digital addiction is so bad for our performance. Based on recent scientific studies, she compiled a detox programme that can help you drastically reduce your digital touchpoints — all the digital channels and media you use, such as your work e-mail, your private e-mail, WhatsApp, text messages, Instagram and internal company chats.

You start by figuring out where, when and why you use a certain medium (e-mail, text messages, chat) and device (smartphone, tablet). Do you check the news on your tablet? Do you mainly shop online or keep in contact with your relatives via a chat group? After you have got a picture of your digital touchpoints, you can start making choices. For example, you could decide not to read or send any WhatsApp messages after nine in the evening, to schedule two phone-free hours when you can work without interruption or to no longer install certain social media channels on your phone.

What would such a digital detox look like at work? The key is to make the right decisions at the right time. I am not opposed to digitalization but I *am* calling for us to use digitalization in ways that benefit our brains, and therefore our wellbeing. A sound digital policy takes into account when you need to focus (with as little interruption and distraction as possible) and which tasks should be synchronous.

In an ideal world there would be clearly defined focus blocks in your diary, times when you would (usually) be doing asynchronous work. Home is a good place for this kind of work, but some people find they can focus better at the office. These focus blocks work well if you go 'cold turkey' and try to avoid all digital stimulation. If you and your colleagues do asynchronous work, it is also important to take one another's focus blocks into account. It is a good idea to inform them when you have scheduled focus time, just as it is useful for you to know when the colleagues in your team don't want to be disturbed. A shared digital diary could be a solution here.

In addition to blocking in time for deep work, you will also need to earmark time for your day-to-day tasks. Choose the appropriate medium. Some things can be dealt with perfectly well by e-mail whereas others are better handled by phone. Try to decide on a specific medium for each type of communication and keep to it. If you get information from a colleague by e-mail, on WhatsApp and through the internal chat system, you will soon lose track of things.

What about meetings? They will require more planning in a hybrid work context. Dynamic, creative topics are best discussed in a meeting where all the team are present in person, sitting around the table. So schedule these meetings at times when everyone is in the office. Informative meetings, status updates and discussions of more technical matters could be done online.

Whether you hold the meeting online or in person, you should always specify at the start how long the meeting will go on for and what you aim to achieve. That is a prerequisite for letting everyone at the meeting get in a flow. The best — and often shortest — meetings are aware ones. Draw up an agenda beforehand and send it to everyone. Think about who could and should be invited, start and stop the meeting on time and spend the last five minutes summarizing it. Keep all the attendees involved and energized. You can do that for example by regularly asking for feedback, addressing attendees directly, using different people to write the minutes and keeping eye contact.

Consider alternative forms of communication too. Before you plan a video call, ask yourself whether you really need to hold a meeting about this topic. If so, what can you do to make sure you spend the meeting time profitably? You can send your team a lot of information beforehand, and thereby reduce the time needed to agree matters in the meeting itself (whether online or offline). An example is data reports: you can send them to people before the meeting, they can read the report at their leisure and then ask any specific questions during the meeting. That is far more inspiring than spending the first half hour all staring at an Excel spreadsheet full of numbers.

Create rituals

Earlier in this book, I discussed how routines and rituals can give you something to hold onto (see page 95). I get in focus by listening to Leonard Cohen. If I want to really concentrate on a task, I listen to his song *Take This Waltz*. The moment I hear the first few notes, my brain gets a signal: watch out, you are about to focus hard on a task. The rhythm automatically sweeps me up in a flow.

An employee of one of our clients told me that she used to work on the kitchen table during the pandemic. But she did not just shove the breakfast things to one side when she began her working day. Instead, she spread out a special tablecloth in a different colour as her own personal ritual for starting the day. That is an excellent idea. Make sure you create a transition from your private life to your work. Replace your daily commute with a short walk, or a cup of coffee in the garden or on the balcony. You can incorporate rituals during the working day too. For example, you could move to another room or switch music channels when you change from one task to the next. Perhaps a strong beat is just the thing to urge you on with administrative tasks, and perhaps you are better able to answer e-mails when standing upright. And don't forget to remove the tablecloth at the end of the afternoon so you finish the working day with a ritual too.

Be authentic

The crisis cut through our physical connections with our co-workers but unexpectedly brought more togetherness and cohesion than ever before. "I now know quite a few people who I've been working very closely with during this past year and who I've never met in person. People who now know me quite well and I know them quite well, but I have never seen their legs... though I've seen their homes, kids and pets." This was Danish graphic designer Mona Ebdrup's apt description of the situation on Twitter.

During the pandemic, we got to know our colleagues in a different, more authentic way. That authenticity was an antidote to the isolation in which we found ourselves. Jared Spataro, Corporate Vice-President at Microsoft 365, put it like this: "Before the pandemic, we encouraged people to 'bring their whole self to work,' but it was tough to truly empower them to do that. The shared vulnerability of this time has given us a huge opportunity to bring real authenticity to company culture and transform work for the better." Now we started and ended our e-mails with personal updates, wishes and questions, while digital meetings gave us a glimpse of our colleagues' home lives. A survey by Microsoft revealed that 18 per cent of the respondents had 'met' their co-workers' pets or families online and that 17 per cent had shed some tears with a colleague. That figure was even higher in the sectors that suffered most from the pandemic (20 per cent in education, 21 per cent in travel and tourism, and 23 per cent in the health services). 39 per cent of people felt they could be themselves more at work and 31 per cent felt less ashamed if aspects of their private lives became known at work.

And that is good news! People who are in close contact with their colleagues not only have stronger work relationships, they are also more productive and enjoy superior wellbeing. Authentic personal interactions have the power to foster inclusion and innovation.

I have long been in favour of people consciously revealing their authentic selves at work. Before COVID-19, I often saw people behaving totally differently at work compared with in private. It was as if they had a work personality and a private personality. But that is ridiculous: we are one person. I like to call this work-life integration. If you always present your true identity and are upfront about your 'why' and your values, in the final analysis you will have more energy. To be sure, you may find this authentic you is not to the liking of some people, but others will be all the more enthusiastic.

This vulnerability can be incredibly powerful. For example, when I was going through my divorce I would sometimes tell my colleagues on a Monday about how difficult I had found the weekend without the kids. By being honest, I didn't waste energy on pretending I had had a great weekend. It also meant that my colleagues would understand without me having to be explicit why I had worked for a couple of hours on the Sunday and why I wanted to leave on time on the Monday to pick up the children. My own honesty also encouraged colleagues to do the same. They regularly opened up without shame about their lives. Not only did we become familiar with one another's home decor, we got to know one another better as people, and that strengthened our bonds.

A hybrid career

"I've found that working remotely has given me more space for long-term thinking and helped me spend more time with my family, which has made me happier and more productive at work," wrote Facebook CEO Mark Zuckerberg in early June 2021 in an internal memo. He immediately allowed full-time staff at the social media company to continue working remotely for another six months at least. I should emphasize that this announcement was a major U-turn. In May 2020, staff were told that only experienced employees would be given permission to work from home.

The Facebook CEO's message contains certain keywords that show he had realized how a focus on hybrid work could give him a competitive advantage. Those keywords are 'long-term thinking' and 'more productive' but also 'family' and 'happier'. It is good to see that he wants his employees to benefit from this competitive advantage too. Although at present many managers have no choice but to take their workers' individual wishes into account for financial reasons. The days when people lived for their job are gone. We are still willing to invest in our careers and building a productive and impactful working life, but we are no longer prepared to do so at the expense of our personal happiness. If you no longer identify with your employer, you go and work for the competition, or in an industry or company where mental wellbeing and hybrid work *are* taken seriously. Mark Zuckerberg has understood that only too well. If he did not allow hybrid work, it was highly likely that many Facebook staff — who have a strong position in the labour market — would jump ship sooner or later.

And they would be quite right to do so! Why should you spend your entire life working for the same employer? Why let your career be determined by chance developments and opportunities? Why should your choice of university degree at the age of 18 determine your career, and why should your work be a part-time or full-time job? Time to consciously craft your career!

THE TRANSITION PERIOD

The coronavirus crisis let many of us take a step back and gave us the time to think hard about how we wanted to work in the future, not only on a day-to-day basis but also in the longer term. Many people started to reflect on their jobs and their lives, on the choices they had made and their central 'why'. Rightly so.

Any crisis — and that includes a global pandemic — is a call to action for you not just as a person, but also as an employee or freelancer. Now is the time to weigh up the pros and cons of your current situation. What works for you and what doesn't? What makes you productive and happy, and what doesn't? Where do you need a mental reset?

Instigating a reset in your work is a process of brainstorming, working out a plan, trying it out and evaluating. That process is just as important as the result. Don't just automatically adopt that standard 'three days in the office, two days at home' approach. Figure out what works for *you* in your current circumstances. Try out new solutions, discuss them with your employer, tell them how it's going, ask for feedback and evaluate. Anthropologist Jitske Kramer advocates extending the period of doubt: don't commit to a particular solution straight away, continue experimenting until you can be sure what is right for *you*. She talks literally about "prolonging the discomfort" so that you can explore what place work has in your life. We must resist the temptation to cast our new way of working in a rigid mould. We are better off extending the transition period, the 'meanwhile' that we are currently in, rather than trying to make decisions too quickly. After all, people are most open to new options in such a transition period. Just as new plant species evolve in the transitional zone between two biotopes, so the most innovative ideas emerge when we are undergoing change. So give yourself permission to vacillate. That does not mean doing nothing or taking a wait-and-see attitude; it means daring to experiment without yet taking a final decision. Because what applies to companies — namely that they are in a 'test and learn' phase — applies equally and above all to you as an individual.

TAKE OWNERSHIP OF YOUR OWN CAREER

How do you instigate a career reset? You can start by asking yourself questions at the macro level. Where do I want my future to be headed? What place do I want my job to have in my life? What energizes me? Which talents do I want to make use of? Do I use my talents enough in my current job? Does my job address my 'why'? Does my current position offer me enough opportunities for growth? Am I getting a chance to specialize or do courses? Is my work good for my wellbeing? Do I feel safe mentally? Am I given the chance to try things out, fail, learn from that and try again?

Drawing up a hybrid career path for yourself also means incorporating flexibility that allows for the different stages in your lifecycle. Are you a young parent or have your children already left home? Do you temporarily need to spend more time on health issues, whether your own or those of a relative?

To figure out at the micro level how to integrate working from home in your job, you need to ask yourself the following questions. At what times and in what places was I most productive? Which tasks did I do then and how much satisfaction did I get from completing these tasks or taking on certain responsibilities? Are there tasks I can get done more quickly at home than at the office? What working hours are most productive for me? Do I get as much energy from face-to-face meetings as from video-call meetings?

Look for broader weekly or monthly patterns. You could also set up a trial period for yourself and your employer to find the right balance for you between productivity and personal welfare.

A HUMAN CAPITAL SCAN

I regularly perform what I term a 'human capital scan' for companies that want to prevent burnout and increase staff welfare at work. We use surveys and data to measure the factors that generate stress or energy in the company. Is there role-related stress; do employees in a particular position know which responsibilities they can or must adopt? What are the digital stress levels? Is there an internal policy for answering e-mails and chat messages? Are all employees reachable in the evenings and weekends? What is expected of them in that regard?

The scan is partly an analysis of the risk factors that could threaten staff wellbeing but it also identifies the opportunities – the human capital and the energizing factors. What makes the employees happy, what talents do they have and what results do they want to achieve? How can they perform at their best?

In the past, the report of the scan would just have gone to the management but now the staff get to read it too. That gives them the chance to take ownership and implement the tips from the report in their jobs. That in turn increases their resilience, agility, autonomy and engagement. I have seen employees in a company where the scan showed a high risk of burnout take the initiative to change the corporate culture from the bottom up. They stopped sending one another e-mails in the evening, introduced lunchtime walking and jogging groups and made agreements with one another about focus time. The scan was a wake-up call and they felt a joint responsibility to respond.

NURTURE A GROWTH MINDSET

Drone operator, investor in bitcoins, 3D printer maintenance engineer. No one who graduated from college more than ten years ago could have done a course preparing them for these job vacancies in 2021. Hybrid work also means diversifying. Your career is not set in stone from day one, and this reset won't be your last. The days in which we could work for the same company our entire lives, do the same job, or even be sure that our current profession would still exist in three years are long gone. That is why lifelong learning has increasingly become the norm. It is important to adopt that mindset of lifelong learning. Not only will it increase your employability and options in the jobs market, it will also give you more personal satisfaction. After all, being able to develop determines our happiness at work.

In *Mindset. The New Psychology of Success,* Stanford professor Carol Dweck discusses the results of her years of research on people's self-image. How people describe themselves has a big impact on how they work, learn and interact with others, and consequently on the rest of their lives. She says the distinction can be summarized by two extremes: the fixed mindset and the growth mindset. People with a fixed mindset assume all their qualities are fixed whereas people with a growth mindset are convinced that they can learn anything with enough time and effort. The fixed-mindset people find feedback scary and see successful people as a threat. The growth-mindset people love feedback and they observe successful people to learn from them.

The working environment is often full of factors that encourage a fixed mindset: people or processes standing in the way of your growth aspirations or innovative ideas. For example, you get turned down every time you ask if you can do an extra course. Or nothing is done with your idea for making various day-to-day business processes more efficient. Or there is no room for drawing up a strategy for long-term change in your department. In companies with a growth mindset, on the other hand, information is shared eagerly, managers are keen on innovation and there is a culture of giving feedback and encouraging staff to collaborate and learn from their mistakes.

To nurture a growth mindset, you need to identify the triggers of a fixed mindset and learn how to deal with them. Think about yourself for a moment. How do you respond to challenges? What do you do when faced with obstacles? How much effort do you currently put into learning something new? How do you deal with criticism? What is your reaction when others are successful? Do you see yourself as work in progress, someone who is always willing and able to learn?

See the clip about the growth mindset
on the Mental Reset video channel.

Having a growth mindset is essential if you want to implement a successful work reset and embrace hybrid working. This brings to mind one of our clients, an accountancy firm. When you enter their car park, you see a sign saying 'growth mindset: this way' and 'fixed mindset: turn around'. That says it all. That is a company where experimenting and trying out new approaches to work is embedded in the culture. We were already working with this company on mental capital before the pandemic, so the staff had a solid basis in terms of resilience. When people were first permitted to return to the office in small groups after the strict lockdown, the mindset was positive, as could be expected. The personnel were open to change. Yet the employees soon found that the connection with one another was not what they had hoped, as everyone was at the office at different times. So after a couple of weeks, the firm's HR officers worked out a different solution for the new system. Now colleagues in the same team could see one another, but the timetable was completely different to the original solution. I had expected some resistance at first. After all, you are asking the team to make yet another change. But it went well, and the staff responded enthusiastically. The resilience of this firm's staff and their ability to cope flexibly with the changes after the pandemic were greater precisely because this company had already invested in a growth mindset and mental wellbeing before the crisis.

GIVE YOUR CAREER OXYGEN THROUGHOUT YOUR LIFE

"I believe life-long learning is key," says Lynda Gratton, professor of Management Practice at London Business School. She adds, "The traditional concept of a 'three-stage life', made up of three distinct periods of full-time education, full-time working, and then full-time retirement, is clearly untenable over a long life. How could a one-shot investment in learning be sufficient for a working life that stretches over 60 years — and that takes place during a time of profound technological disruption? A more future-proofed concept is a 'multistage life', in which learning and education are distributed across the whole of a lifetime."

There has already been a clear change for the better in the past few years, with incentives for career counselling and more companies providing staff with in-house and external training. But why should employees limit themselves to these traditional options when they can also independently make use of a global offering online? Why should you wait until your employer gives you permission to do a course when you can proactively oxygenate your brain and your career? Joris, an old school friend of mine who had a degree in Communication Science, was constantly running into problems because he didn't meet the demanding IT requirements for the jobs he was interested in. So he started doing online courses to rectify that. Over the past few years he has mastered four programming languages and explored machine learning and artificial neural networks. Now he is a much sought-after data scientist who builds robots in his free time. "People sometimes ask me whether I regret my choice of degree subject," says Joris. "I don't hold with that. Online courses let me become whatever I want to be. At the moment I'm thinking about taking up investment so I'm looking for a course that is up to date and covers aspects such as cryptocurrencies."

The online courses Joris is talking about are the Massive Open Online Courses (MOOCs). MIT, Stanford, Harvard and Berkeley were among the first to offer these MOOCs and other organizations soon followed suit. You can currently choose from a huge range of modules all over the world, from an introduction to psychology, genetics or sustainability to courses on cryptography, data mining or artificial intelligence. Worldwide, around 70 million people are studying via the leading MOOC platforms Coursera, edX and FutureLearn. It is interesting to note that LinkedIn acquired the learning platform Lynda.com in 2015. It was able to use its data on job vacancies and learning capacity to offer 9,000 digital courses to 450 million people. "This partnership alone creates huge possibilities for new data-driven, personalized learning paths. This is an exciting, rapidly disrupting sector," says Professor Lynda Gratton.

Online learning has a long way to go — many students complain that there is little to no personal interaction and average completion rates are low (around 10 per cent) — but the potential is huge. It lets employees oxygenate their new hybrid careers throughout their lives and that is a development I can only applaud.

PIXELLATED WORKFORCE

More and more people are working as freelancers, and platform-economy companies such as Uber and Deliveroo are booming. The idea that a job is a single full-time or part-time assignment was already crumbling before the pandemic. In the United States, 42 per cent of workers under the age of 35 are freelancers. People there are more likely to work on a project basis, a results basis or by the hour. In other words, their tasks and achievements are the determining factor, not their position. HR specialist Josh Bersin calls this "the pixellated workforce". Each individual is a separate, independent worker who can be engaged by a company as a pixel. If you want to upgrade your company's website, you could hire someone full-time. But for a temporary, creative project like this, it could be more efficient to engage a part-time consultant, bring in a design company or even get a team based on the other side of the world working online on the task.

Workers in the gig economy also stand to benefit from hybrid work. In the past, freelancers sometimes complained that they were not properly involved by the company hiring them, while employers accused them of a lack of engagement. Now that permanent employees are also working from home, the distinction between them and the freelancers has blurred. It is no longer so clear in mixed teams who the freelancers are and who the employees are. I am therefore expecting 'pixellization' to really take off after the pandemic. Large numbers of people will take ownership of their careers.

A reset is teamwork

CAMPFIRE MOMENTS

At the start of the Covid crisis, employees and team members felt a strong sense of solidarity with one another. The source of this solidarity was their shared vulnerability. They were afraid of the virus and were in an unprecedented situation. As I discussed earlier, that common vulnerability and associated authenticity generated a bond between colleagues and managers.

Yet we also felt we were missing something. We discovered that the office, in whatever form, was a good place to meet up, brainstorm, take action quickly and collaborate productively. That office does not need to be a large building in a city centre. A regional hub, a co-working space, a flexible workspace and meeting room at a train station or on an arterial road can all be good alternatives to the cramped workstations and open-plan offices that we have long known are disastrous for our productivity.

During the coronavirus crisis, the Boston Consulting Group's Henderson Institute held a survey among 12,000 professionals in the United States, Germany and India. The most surprising result was the outsize impact of social connectivity on productivity. Employees who said they were satisfied with the social ties with their colleagues were two to three times more productive in their collaboration than the employees who were dissatisfied with the connectivity. This shows that social connectivity is what enables us to work together productively. It helps us communicate better, work more efficiently, learn faster and be more innovative.

We are in essence incredibly social creatures. Our relationships with others are crucial to our trust, safety and creativity. Anything that undermines that sense of connection affects our resilience. We want to be part of our social tribe, but the pandemic disrupted that belonging. We no longer had our 'campfire moments', the minutes after a meeting when you are in contact with your colleagues, and that meant an end to what organizational psychologists call transformational interactions — the interactions that create the organization's distinct culture. You don't get such transformational interactions in an online meeting where you run through a project plan in a series of bullet points, but you do in informal encounters or meetings designed to create engagement. Anthropologist Jitske Kramer says these interactions tend to be the times when people genuinely listen to one another and are prepared to change their opinions. In other words, the moments when change happens.

So hybrid work also needs to allow room for such campfire moments. They happen spontaneously when you are at the office, but when working online you will need to deliberately schedule such "useful superfluity", as Professor Steven Poelmans of the Antwerp Management School called these moments in an interview. "'Useful superfluity' is good for creating bonds. These are moments that seem superfluous but are actually necessary: the chatter between meetings or when getting a coffee. If I have a virtual meeting, I log in a bit early. You can also invite other people to do so and then you can have a chat first. You can do the same at the end, to let people talk to one another afterwards. A big mistake I often see is scheduling back-to-back meetings with no time in between. Leave some buffers."

The coronavirus crisis has finally put paid to a major taboo, namely mental health problems. Now we were all facing challenges to our mental health, whether we were factory workers or managers, pupils or teachers, employees or freelancers. The chronic uncertainty and the oscillating restrictions and relaxations forced us to dig deep into our mental reserves.

How did organizations try to maintain the productive social network of colleagues and team members during the health crisis? How did they make sure that team members could find one another and support and encourage each other? In some companies, one-on-one conversations online with managers worked wonders. Other organizations deliberately tried to coach the remote workers in setting limits. Some staff organized digital coffee breaks, online update sessions, rounds of questions, TGIF zoom sessions on Friday evenings or meetings combined with a walk.

There is no single proven recipe for creating or maintaining team spirit. However, certain key principles or tips can be identified. One is that you must not add to the digital overload in the name of mental welfare. That means no online quiz if your staff have spent the entire day in online meetings. And no compulsory online social drinks event just when the kids get home from school, because that simply deprives your employees of the benefits of working from home.

A proper staff welfare policy must be more than an annual team-building session. It is all very well having a bunch of flowers delivered to an employee's home, but if that is not part of a joined-up policy, it will have no more effect than the basket of fruit that was *de rigueur* in the office in days gone by. We are noticing the shift at Better Minds at Work, where we have seen a big increase in the demand for training relating to mental welfare.

Welfare at work is no longer an empty slogan; it has become a key issue for managers. Companies that dismissed this as 'unnecessary' in the past now have no alternative but to jump on the bandwagon. In the future, employees will ask what coaching, mental health counselling or welfare monitoring their employer offers. And rightly so. The pandemic has shown that there is a clear association between mental health and productivity.

CHAPTER 5

THE MOST HYBRID EMPLOYER OF THE YEAR

A NEW ERA REQUIRES NEW LEADERS

Leadership in hybrid times

"We have to take 100 per cent of the decisions with 50 per cent of the knowledge." This statement by the Dutch prime minister Mark Rutte may ring true for many senior managers. Managers too have to steer their ships through mist.

Crises are a test of leadership, giving strong leaders a chance to shine while poor leaders have nowhere to hide. If you are a director, head of a department, manager or team supervisor, you undoubtedly learned new things about your staff during the pandemic, and probably about yourself too. How did you deal with the uncertainty? Were you honest and respectful in your treatment of your employees? Did you go through a moaning phase, or were you able to adapt quickly and give your employees the aids and assistance they needed?

Trust is an essential concept for managers whose teams are working remotely. Strong leaders inspire their staff by communicating with them regularly and demonstrating empathy. This makes the employees feel safe. But good leaders are also visionaries who are prepared to go against the tide. They keep an open mind and embrace diversity.

Good leadership in hybrid times is challenging but also offers real opportunities for growth. After all, these leaders will be the ones who can attract and retain the outstanding international workers.

THE CHIEF EMPATHY OFFICER

"Companies are hiring Chief Health Officers, Head of Safety and Wellbeing, and Directors of Wellbeing like never before. In fact, there are 55,000 jobs now open for Directors of Wellbeing, VPs of

Wellbeing, or Wellbeing managers in business. CEO now means Chief Empathy Officer," argues Josh Bersin in *The Secret to Wellbeing at Work is... Leadership*.

Before the health crisis, managers never approached me with a request for a session on employee engagement, but for the past few months demand for this service has been booming. It is as if managers discovered *en masse* during the pandemic that engagement and productivity are closely interlinked. At Better Minds at Work, we organize special break-out sessions in which managers and team leaders learn how to connect with their team based on questions about emotions and wellbeing. We train them in listening, flexibility and a caring attitude — in other words, in empathy.

The first thing I tell people in workshops is that empathic leaders need to focus on the internal situation. The Chief Empathy Officer of the year is not someone who spends their whole time promoting an image of their company to the outside world as a great place to work. On the contrary, they increase staff wellbeing by demonstrating empathy.

I regularly point to the three key factors determining happiness at work: autonomy, involvement and competence. We know these three factors increase our job satisfaction. Leaders who put these principles into practice will find it easier to motivate their team and keep them happy. To put it another way, they are empathically proactive. What do autonomy, involvement and competence mean when work is hybrid? Let me give some pointers.

→ AUTONOMY. Working from home gave many employees a high degree of autonomy. That was welcome for people who had been doing their job for a while but could be stressful for new employees. Empathic leaders are alert to that distinction and make sure that all employees have the necessary tools to operate autonomously on the days they work from home. Or they let new employees who struggle with the autonomy come to the office more often than other staff.

- → INVOLVEMENT. I have already discussed the consequences of hybrid work for our social contacts at work and elsewhere at some length. Here too, employees will vary in the extent to which they find this a problem. Someone who is new to the job, lives alone and does not have a wide social network in their private life may find one day at the office is not enough to satisfy their needs, whereas someone with a family, a large circle of friends and a strong professional network may feel this is sufficient. Your task as an empathic leader is to encourage engagement and take your employees' differing needs into account when drawing up new work arrangements.
- → COMPETENCE. The most important precondition for happiness at work is the ability to grow. As a leader, you should ask yourself how do your employees learn. Do they do it formally or informally? Formal training can take place online in some sectors, but informal learning is most effective in the form of live interaction. So you should make sure that employees who can learn from one another are in the office at the same time.

BE A 'DON'T KNOW'

When Amy Edmondson, professor of Leadership and Management at Harvard Business School, studied successful teams in the medical sector, she came to a surprising conclusion. She discovered a clear relationship between the success of different teams within the same company and the number of mistakes they made: the more successful a team was, the more mistakes they made. How was that possible? Edmondson delved into the phenomenon, did some additional research and came up with a correction to her initial conclusion. Successful teams don't necessarily make more mistakes but they do talk about them more. They can speak out freely, including to their manager, without fearing loss of face or being branded incompetent. That is not something that can be taken for granted. Edmondson identified three conditions that need to be satisfied to create psychological safety.

FRAME THE WORK

We need to change how we look at success in work. Failure and mistakes need to be normalized. The response of Toyota director Fujio Cho when one of his employees boasted about the achievements of that week is legendary. "I know you're a good manager," said Cho. "Otherwise we wouldn't have hired you. But please tell me about your problems so that we can find a solution together."

ASK GOOD QUESTIONS

Don't behave like someone who knows everything. Be modest and act like a 'don't know'. Ask questions such as "What is not going well?" or "Who has a different perspective?" or "What signs are we missing?" Proactively asking good questions is the only way you can pick up signals at an early stage that point to potential problems on the horizon.

RESPOND PRODUCTIVELY

If someone brings you bad news, start by saying "Thank you", followed by "How can we help?" That shows your appreciation and shifts the focus on the future straight away. You only turn your attention to the causes later.

It basically all comes down to the same message: try, fail, learn and repeat. As a leader, you must give your staff room to try things out and to fail. It is important that they are allowed to learn from their failure and make another attempt. In short, there is a strong link between growth and success on the one hand and being able and willing to fail on the other. As the great basketball player Michael Jordan said, "I've missed more than 9,000 shots in my career. I've lost almost 300 games. Twenty-six times, I've been trusted to take the game-winning shot and missed. I've failed over and over and over again in my life. And that is why I succeed."

But all too often in my experience, if an employee tries something new and the first results are unsatisfactory, the manager will take the task out of the employee's hands. "It will be easier if I take over," I hear them say. But the employee needs to learn how to overcome the issues themselves. Only then will they experience having learned something. Only then can they reinforce their growth mindset.

For example, one of our speakers told me a week before he was due to give an important talk that he had been struggling with stage fright since the start of the pandemic. He suggested to me that it might be better if a colleague were to take over the session, as he didn't want to ruin the talk. Of course, this was an unpleasant surprise for me as the CEO, but I never considered replacing him for even one fraction of a second. If I didn't place my trust in him now, his stage fright would only grow further. So instead I asked him how we could help him as a team. The other colleagues seated around the table were also very understanding. Someone else shared the fact that she had suffered similar problems, while others gave him tips on how they control their nerves. Everyone stayed surprisingly down to earth. And just being able to tell people what he was going through seemed to lift a burden off his shoulders. Because I put my trust in him, I implicitly also gave him the message that he was allowed to fail. That, in combination with the tips from his co-workers, turned out to be enough to make his talk a success.

I am however pleased to see the taboo among managers on sharing stories of failure is in decline. When I attended network events a decade ago, I would routinely hear managers boasting about their achievements. If the conversation took a turn in that direction, I soon lost interest. Not much can be learned from the successes of others because – like Tolstoy's happy families –success stories are all alike. Nowadays, there is often an explicit announcement at the start of such events that anything we share will remain within the room. And that works: I hear less boasting and more honest revelations.

IT NEVER SIMPLY BLOWS OVER

During the first few weeks and months of the coronavirus crisis, I met managers who thought it would all blow over. After a pause of say six months, we would return to business as usual. That was also their message to their staff, which only meant their employees had to cope with an extra setback when it became clear that Covid was going to be affecting our lives and work for much longer.

Other leaders in contrast proved to be true visionaries, in my eyes. They looked for opportunities, questioned old habits and were prepared to sketch a different roadmap for their team.

In times of crisis, we need visionary leaders, department heads, team supervisors or managers who feel comfortable in a culture of permanent change and who can offer their team the prospect of an inviting future. After all, a crisis like this makes many employees feel insecure. Take the digital transformation that has been underway for some time but was ramped up several gears during the pandemic. More and more jobs are being automated. That is no reason to panic, as we will get at least as many new jobs in return, but at present staff don't yet know what skills they will need for these new jobs. And that is giving many people a sense of insecurity. Visionary leaders are able to deal with that feeling by taking a proactive approach and drawing up a future-proof route with and for their team or company.

DIFFERENT IS BETTER

All too often I hear team leaders say, "Great, I've found someone who's a perfect match to start work in our team!" At first sight, it seems a good idea to hire people who 'fit in'. But the end result is that your team will be full of people with similar profiles. Even minor changes or challenges can be too much for such a team, as they all have the same frame of reference and identical blind spots and will therefore all come up with the same solution. It seems obvious to me that if you are a leader who wants a successful reset, you will need to focus on inclusion and diversity.

For innovation, you as a leader and your organization need individuals who bring a different perspective, a different set of values and a different background. They will increase the cognitive diversity in your company and broaden rather than consolidate your corporate culture. If your team harbours a diversity of opinions, skills and fields of knowledge, then your organization will be more robust and able to cope with crisis-induced change.

That is also why profiles that combine 'hard' skills such as IT with 'soft' skills such as communications, marketing or management will be much in demand in the future. For the same reason, more attention should be paid in recruitment to the candidate's growth mindset and potential rather than just their academic qualifications or credentials. It can also be useful to put together a team that includes radically different approaches based not only on members' degree subjects but also on their socioeconomic and cultural backgrounds. For example, I always make sure I have a good mix of different age groups if I am putting together a team at Better Minds at Work to prepare a new workshop for a company. That helps us tailor our product to the target group. My 50-year-old colleague is often better able to relate to more senior staff, but she also has more affinity than I do with people in their twenties — after all, she has two children in that age group at home. I also make sure there is always at least one man present in such brainstorm sessions; too often, mental welfare is the domain of women.

Drawing up a policy for hybrid work

You have now learned that flexibility, connectivity and authenticity increase productivity. How can your company or institution make use of that knowledge? In my opinion, there is one golden rule: don't just sit there, get to work on a hybrid work policy!

YOUR COMPANY'S DNA

Drawing up a policy for hybrid work requires a flexible mindset. There is no simple one size fits all. And telling your staff they can work from home one, two or three days a week does not constitute a robust hybrid-work policy. A great deal of thought needs to go into the policy before it can be rolled out. You should see the reset as a chance to review thoroughly all aspects of how your work is organized. Lynda Gratton shows you how to start off in her guide on *How to Do Hybrid Right.*

"Start by identifying key jobs and tasks, determine what the drivers of productivity and performance are for each, and think about the arrangements that would serve them best. Engage employees in the process, using a combination of surveys, personas, and interviews to understand what they really want and need. Think expansively and creatively, with an eye to eliminating duplication and unproductive elements in your current work arrangements. Communicate broadly. Train leaders to manage hybrid teams, and invest in the tools of coordination that will help your teams align their schedules. Finally, ask yourself whether your new hybrid arrangements, whatever they are, accentuate your company's values and support its culture."

That last sentence is particularly important. A hybrid work policy starts with the 'why'! What is the company's mission and how can hybrid work support that mission? Then there is the nature of the work. Some sectors such as government, banking and professional services are well suited to hybrid work and were already experimenting before the pandemic with one day a week working from home. But these sectors were also surprised by the speed at which their staff were able to switch to working remotely and were able to do so much more from home than had originally been thought. There was a real sense of urgency and the presumed obstacles failed to materialize. Online meetings became the new normal, collaborating on documents online a must and recruiting clients online an opportunity.

However, hybrid work is not feasible in some sectors. The Dutch microchip machinery manufacturer ASML for example mainly employs engineers. While you might think they would be able to adopt a highly hybrid work pattern, that is not the case. The engineers have to be on site for the company's core business of building microchip-making equipment, and can only spend 20 per cent of their time working from home.

Drawing up a policy for hybrid work also means that as a company you need to analyse and perhaps improve your work processes. I am using the term 'work processes' to mean not only how the work is organized but also the decision-making culture, the way the company approaches communications and the HR policy, to mention just a few aspects. Onboarding of new employees, measuring team members' output, rolling out new decisions and internal communications, for example, may all need to be revised. You will also need to review practical aspects such as the insurance situation for people working at home or on site. And perhaps you will need to purchase new tools to facilitate hybrid meetings, or reconsider staff benefits.

It also means you will need to make new agreements on all these aspects with your staff. Because, as HR specialist Josh Bersin says, "There is no management by walking around anymore." The organization's HR philosophy needs to have solid foundations. If the agreements with staff were already on shaky ground before Covid, you will not be able to draw up a consistent framework of arrangements on hybrid work and get people to keep to them. You will need to work on those foundations first.

If you have a transparent work structure and division of tasks that is accepted by your workforce, you are essentially also fostering the welfare and mental health of your staff. During the pandemic, we have all seen how people's resilience and mental agility came under pressure from all the unanticipated changes in epidemiological, professional and social terms. As an employer, you should therefore avoid adding to this with an unclear or unpredictable protocol on hybrid work. Explain clearly and concisely why and when arrangements will change.

That does not mean you should introduce changes overnight; far from it. As George Anders of LinkedIn puts it bluntly, "Be prepared to draw up a new plan — not once but perhaps two, three, four times. What worked for your people and company in April might not be the same as what works in November." According to him, the best CEOs "will be constantly reassessing the balance between caution and enthusiasm, which will undoubtedly shift in the course of 2021."

The choices that companies and other organizations make now will affect their productivity and their ability to compete for the most talented workers. You should therefore leave room for doubt, experiments and pilot projects. The health crisis has offered companies a unique opportunity to create an inclusive and authentic corporate culture and in doing so, improve performance. You should not be too quick to conclude you have a finished product; keep going until your policy works well for all stakeholders.

A CONVERSATION STARTER

In the summer of 2021, I found a message in my inbox from a concerned acquaintance. His charismatic and successful employer in the entertainment business had drawn up a new company charter for his staff. On his own, without any kind of consultation. The charter stated that all staff were required to come into the office on Mondays, Wednesdays and Fridays. The new policy caused an uproar. From a business operations perspective, having those days as office days made sense and was quite justifiable. But by that point staff had been working their fingers to the bone, so when they had no say in the new policy, there was a great deal of resistance (and rightly so).

It seems like a no-brainer yet people still often fail to take this into account: hybrid work arrangements are not something you can just draw up yourself in between your other tasks. Arriving at that framework is a process that requires internal and external expertise, but also the involvement and input of the staff concerned. Only then will you be able to take decisions that enjoy broad support and can last for several years while also allowing room for flexibility.

Fluvius, a Belgian grid operator for electricity and natural gas, shows how it should be done. In the course of 2021, the company drew up a charter for remote work based on the findings of an internal working group. Then they asked Better Minds at Work to inspire their internal coaches with a presentation and an online session of questions and answers with all kinds of questions being fired off. In the next stage, Better Minds at Work produced a video for each remote working rule in which we clarified the scientific foundation for the rule. We explained how the policy was good for the brain, paying attention to focus, breaks, elephants and rabbits.

Explaining why these remote working rules were needed was crucial in getting staff involved and overcoming any resistance. What is more, the videos functioned as a conversation starter in the teams rather than being presented as a take-it-or-leave-it message. For in addition to the company-wide charter, the individual teams within Fluvius had to come up with agreements specific to that team. Team managers could even tailor arrangements at the individual level. The result was a remote-working charter that had the backing of staff and offered sufficient flexibility.

WHAT AN EMPTY OFFICE MEANS

On Tuesday 13 July 2021, I walked out of the lift into the office of a producer of bottled water. Except for the receptionist who kindly welcomed me and the two employees I was meeting, the entire floor of this large office in Brussels was deserted. It was actually quite worrying. Throughout the COVID-19 crisis, the company's staff had complained bitterly that they were unable to come to the office and as a result felt unable to connect to one another. Now it was possible to return to the head office in person, yet the building was still empty. The responsible managers were at their wits' end? How was that possible? What was going on?

It seemed clear to me that the reason for this resistance lay in too many demands being made of the employees' resilience and a lack of willpower. At that point, most staff had had their resilience tested more than normal for some eighteen months — quite a long time. Their mental energy levels had fallen dramatically. Asking them to perform a work reset at that moment was essentially exposing them to a resilience experiment on top of the previous resilience experiment. The pandemic had sapped their willpower and empathy, such that the primeval human was taking over in them. The primeval human is much quicker to resist change than our rational selves would normally be. Combined with the fact that staff had been taking new brain pathways for eighteen months, this was what was causing the empty offices.

In many organizations, empty offices symbolize the resistance to change. Returning to the office means sitting in traffic jams again, arranging childcare and possibly disrupting the work-life balance again. A survey among our clients showed that employees were afraid they would not be able to concentrate in the office, they would be less productive and would end up having to catch up with work again in the evenings and weekends. They were convinced that the office could only function as a place for meeting up, chatting and brainstorming. They feared that having to come into the office would affect their productivity negatively.

I see two ways to get staff back to the office: reduce the threshold for the change — the return — and increase their resilience.

You can reduce the threshold by making the switch to working in the office a gradual and pleasant process, for example by introducing a 'reboarding' ritual. Some companies have done just that. One example is DPG Media, which gave its staff a football shirt when they returned (see page 38). The return should also be designed to counter any preconceptions your team might have. So make sure your first in-person brainstorm session is a success. Or let staff do work requiring concentration at home first and only come to the office after the rush hour.

Increasing employees' resilience requires an in-depth approach. At Better Minds at Work, we have launched an offering of workshops and lectures aimed at fostering a growth mindset in staff. We did this for the Belgian cable company Telenet, where we showed in detail what hybrid work would look like for everyone in an interactive workshop. Not only did this increase ownership of this new way of working, it also allowed the brain pathways of staff to gradually adjust to the impending work reset. Team members were able to focus on the opportunities associated with a return to the office rather than remaining fixated on resistance.

MICE AT PLAY

"When the cat's away, the mice will play." Unfortunately, that is still how many CEOs and managers see things. They force their staff to come to the office on the assumption that they do not have enough of a work ethic to be equally productive at home.

The HR director of an international manufacturer of plastic gloves told me that when the top man is at the office, all employees without exception make sure they are there too. Being visibly present demonstrates your engagement and your desire for promotion. The boss of the glove company also makes a habit of regularly flying in all the directors for a team meeting. That was not possible for the HR director during the pandemic as she lives in the United Kingdom, which had strict quarantine rules at the time. The director was therefore forced to make a video call, which made her wonder not surprisingly, "What price am I paying for working remotely?"

Sad to say, that is often how it works at major international companies. And we need to put a stop to it. You should not reward or promote employees for being in the right place at the right time and saying the right things to the right people. You should reward them for genuinely adding value to their team and organization. And that can be achieved perfectly well through remote, asynchronous work. A hybrid work policy should put an end to the benefits from 'presenteeism' and make sure substance is rewarded instead.

That means that when you have a hybrid meeting, you open and close the meeting formally, you don't take any new decisions during the lunch with just the people present at that time, and the chair regularly addresses the participants who are attending the meeting by video.

I want to make clear that I am no advocate of invisible, ghostly employees. There needs to be a balance. If you never have any contact with your colleagues and managers, this is likely to have a negative effect in all kinds of areas. In the worst case, you become completely alienated from one another. One example, albeit rather extreme, is of a man who was made redundant by the municipality of Antwerp in 2000. However, he was never sent an official notice of dismissal, so his salary continued to be paid. He said nothing, but neither was he called up by the municipality for five years. When this error finally came to light, he was dismissed for a second time, this time with all the requisite formalities. The municipality's negligence ended in a lawsuit and additional financial compensation for the man in question. What a Kafkaesque situation with an invisible employee! Fortunately it doesn't usually get that extreme, but if employees are never seen at all, you soon end up in a counterproductive vicious circle. Managers no longer assign them tasks, so they start underperforming and end up being given even fewer assignments as a result.

MOST EMPLOYEES ARE DECENT FOLK

When a friend of mine started work at a communications company, on her first day she was given a particularly extensive briefing on the system that she would be using to record her hours. She had previously been accustomed as a freelancer to plan her own work and always met her deadlines without any problems, but now she was required to record every minute. She was allowed

45 minutes for a blog post, she was expected to come up with four Facebook posts an hour, and a client presentation could take 60 minutes. When she had to continue working according to that system during the pandemic — with a toddler at home — she couldn't take it anymore. When she phoned me in tears, I asked her why they had that time recording system. "The manager had had a bad experience in the past with an employee who abused the trust in him," she told me. After the manager found out about that, the company based its entire policy on that one employee who was slacking in the hope to keep a firm grip on things in future. It goes without saying that this strategy was not a great success. In the year my friend worked for the company, one employee after another handed in their resignation.

A new policy for hybrid work is such a fundamental intervention in the organization that it is crucial to base it on the large group of motivated workers rather than the occasional individual slacker. The slackers will always find a way to cut corners, but most people are decent folk. More specifically, most employees are decent folk. Most employees have a solid work ethic, want to do valuable, meaningful work, want to see results and want to make an impact. A hybrid work policy should be based on that motivated majority. And because autonomy increases happiness at work, they should be trusted.

We also urgently need to stop obsessing about how many hours people put in. All too often, we have a tendency to tell everyone how busy, busy, busy we are at work. Being reachable at all times — including outside working hours at home — seems to offer proof to your employer or client of how valuable you are. But we don't become more productive by working longer hours — far from it. If we spend too long staring at our computer screens in endless video calls, we find it harder to stay focused and our energy levels fall. It is not the quantity that matters but the quality.

NURTURE YOUR CREATIVE CAPITAL

Too often managers say, "I don't have any use for creative types." In fact, the opposite is true. In future, computers will increasingly take over the non-creative tasks. Artificial intelligence already offers a solution for many repetitive operational tasks. You no longer need humans to enter invoices in your accountancy software, transcribe a sound recording or compile a repayment schedule. What remains are the creative jobs that can only be done by humans. A good accountant is not necessarily the one who knows all the rules inside out, a good secretary is not necessarily the one who can type out the meeting minutes the fastest and a good banker is not the one who can calculate the most favourable repayment schedule. In modern organizations, creative capital in the form of creative employees is the most important resource.

Even more so in a crisis when you need people who can think outside the box, even in the traditionally non-creative departments. Esfan Eghtessadi, commercial director of the fashion label Essentiel, decided that the creative team should also be invited to the crisis meetings during the pandemic. "In retrospect, that was enriching for both sides," says Inge Onsea, the label's creative director. "That cross-fertilization produced innovative ideas. For example, we decided to supply our collections in two stages. It meant the shops didn't have to pay for everything at once and we could also divide the production costs in two. It made things more financially viable for everyone. Incidentally, we sent the second delivery by train or boat, which is much cheaper and more sustainable than by plane. That would have been unthinkable in the past."

So there is a use for creative types. These are precisely the employees who come up with innovations, new products and services and solutions to problems. They are the ones who think ahead and can imagine a visionary future. If you want to innovate, you need people like this. And if you really want to be a pioneer you should not only search actively for new employees who can think creatively but also encourage creative ideas from all the staff in your company and establish an environment that fosters inventiveness.

A well-known example is Google, where staff are given one day a week to work on a creative project of their choosing. Then there is the quote by Bill Gates that he always chooses someone lazy for the most difficult tasks because "a lazy person will find an easy way to do it". Closer to home, Mieke Neven, CEO of the Belgian printing company Burocad, asked everyone in her team for ideas at the start of the pandemic. "I used two criteria to assess the ideas: there needed to be a prototype within one day and it should require an investment of less than a thousand euros. After all, you need to get your ideas on the market as soon as possible at the start of a crisis. You can't sit there at the drawing board until your idea is perfect; you make adjustments afterwards based on the feedback. Do or die!" she explained in an interview with the Belgian magazine *POMblad.* One of the employees discovered at the start of the pandemic that the protective layer under the flag fabric that they printed designs on was suitable for producing facemasks. One month later, Burocad had the requisite certification and was selling hundreds of thousands of facemasks.

In short, cherish the people in your organization who can see beyond the day-to-day concerns (the rabbits), who are good at abstract thinking, who have a perceptive overview of your sector and can link this to realistic objectives.

A CUSTOMIZED COMPANY CHARTER

If you want to make agreements with your team about hybrid work, you will need the concepts I introduced in Chapter 4 concerning flexibility in place (office versus home) and time (synchronous versus asynchronous).

The advantage of that framework of concepts for hybrid work is that you can discuss with your team or directors which dimensions are most important for your team, based on scientific insights. Of course, people's jobs and what they involve can change over time. That means you need to be flexible and adapt the agreements accordingly.

This exercise sounds rather theoretical but it works perfectly well in practice. I can give the example of a European IT company that I advised. Triggered by one of my talks, the head of a large team asked me to help them draw up a new policy for hybrid work. First, Better Minds at Work ran a series of workshops with the employees. After a talk in which we introduced the main concepts, staff were given free rein to think up possibilities for hybrid work. That led to the most exotic proposals. One person suggested working permanently from home and then organizing a two-day meetup for the team once a month at a location that speaks to the imagination. Incidentally, one of the employees took part in the workshop by video-calling from Ibiza. The palm trees in the background were no desktop image — they swayed gently in the breeze. This divergent step, where ideas about hybrid work took off in all directions and nothing was off-limits, was followed by a period of reflection. During this period, the ideas were checked against the concepts. This resulted in a convergent proposal in which various ideas were selected based on what was feasible, desirable and possible within this particular company.

They now have a general charter with clear-cut agreements

at the team and department levels. In other words, they have a framework for hybrid work. Tailored variation is possible for the team and the individual, so that the team can and should respond flexibly to changes in team members' private circumstances. For example, if someone is going through a divorce they can discuss the option of more asynchronous work. Equally, this is possible for someone who needs to work on an assignment requiring more focus.

HYBRID WORK POLICIES IN PRACTICE

Another company that has successfully implemented a hybrid work policy is the accountancy firm PwC. I am not surprised. The Belgian CEO Axel Smits put the welfare of his people front and centre even before the pandemic. From the moment he became CEO in 2016, he prioritized change. Not because change was urgently needed, but because he wanted to keep his staff agile and flexible.

Smits can see the bigger picture, which makes him a visionary. He was already letting his employees work from home even before the government made it compulsory. Nowadays, team members can decide for themselves when and where they work. "Of course this must not be at the expense of the team's cohesion and the service to the client," says Smits. "So I expect most teams will organize meetings at the office, but they don't have to. We also have a stock of virtual tools for fostering the team spirit and letting people work together efficiently." Employees can join a virtual Secret Coffee Break with a member of staff they don't know, and the company provides information on virtual leadership and online brainstorming.

The new PwC campus will also be an activity-based working space, where each area will have a specific function. "A room for focused work should look different to a space where you come up with innovative solutions in a team," says Smits. "We also took employee wellbeing into account in the new layout of the office building. Because employees will need to move around the building depending on the activity, they will get more exercise. We have also created no fewer than nine patios." PwC has chosen an easily accessible location near the airport, aiming to reduce the barrier to coming to the office. "When they were working from home, our staff used what had been commuting time to exercise, do their grocery shopping and so on. Of course we want to minimize that commuting time in the future too," explains Smits.

It is all very interesting, but two aspects in particular struck me. Firstly, the new policy for hybrid work is not a rigid system. "We will refine some things when they are implemented. I am quite sure the policy is not yet tailored to suit all employees and all circumstances." The company will be using regular 'pulse surveys' to get feedback from employees on their findings and requirements. Secondly, PwC is well aware that sound employee welfare is a prerequisite for change. You won't get a growth mindset without resilience. For example, the company has a platform for parents where they can share ideas on the work-life balance, it regularly organizes workshops and inspiration sessions on mental resilience and it offers psychological counselling for anyone who needs it.

It ticks all the boxes. There is flexibility in time and place. And because Smits is a real people person, the brain criterion is the underlying principle determining where and when people work, while the charter itself offers room for change and personal interpretations.

Young employees after the pandemic

One ordinary Wednesday evening, the friends of freelance journalist Eline Van Lancker gather round a bowl of hummus to celebrate the fact that she had resigned after months of wavering. In an article, Eline wrote an 'Ode to the quitters'. She concluded that young people of her generation — who she dubbed the quitter generation — are more likely to say 'no' and choose self-realization, mental wellbeing and the creation of meaningful impact rather than financial rewards. While not everyone has the luxury of being able to head for the exit, she saw young people deciding to chase their dream, their 'why', especially during the pandemic. Friend A started a photography course, friend B moved to an apartment in a co-housing project and friend C rid herself of her relationship, her job and her house in one fell swoop in exchange for a new life in Berlin.

In this chapter, I want to explore the specific situation of young employees during and after the health crisis. On the one hand, young employees faced (and still face) challenges while on the other hand they in particular currently have exceptional opportunities at work. At least, they do if they adopt a growth mindset and go for their 'why'.

A PRECARIOUS SITUATION

Young employees often had a hard time of it during the pandemic. The 2021 Work Trend Index, which combines the results from surveys of more than 30,000 people in 31 countries, shows that Generation Z (aged 18 to 25) was in a precarious position when people had to work remotely. Sixty per cent of the respondents in this generation stated clearly that they were finding it difficult. They are at the start of their careers, are more likely to live on their own and therefore feel the impact of isolation more. They have trouble staying motivated and finding a good work-life balance. They are exhausted after a normal day at work. Members of Generation Z also find it harder to feel engaged, get enjoyment out of their job, speak up during meetings and contribute new ideas.

These figures are not surprising. "Without hallway conversations, chance encounters and small talk over coffee, it's hard to feel connected even to the immediate team, much less build meaningful connections across the company," says Hannah McConnaughey, product marketing manager at Microsoft.

Twenty-seven-year-old Elise also experienced a dip. Elise works for a small non-profit organization, where she was soon given a lot of autonomy for someone her age. She enjoyed this at first, but during the pandemic the autonomy had a paralysing effect. She was barely able to send two e-mails a day from her studio flat. The weekly online meeting with the coordinator did not really energize her either. It was only once she was able to go back into the office in Brussels city centre again for a few days a week that she felt part of team, and was able to breathe freely and be productive again. Just in time.

Mentoring new hires and Generation Z employees when everyone is working remotely is no easy matter. They have yet to build up a network of colleagues within the organization or professional contacts externally who they can call on. What is more, when staff were working from home they started talking more to the colleagues they knew best and trusted, which meant new workers felt even more left out.

New employees faced an additional challenge in the fact that it is particularly difficult to teach new skills via Zoom or Teams. During Covid, they had no opportunity to learn on the job and autonomy is only possible once you have mastered your tasks. Graduate recruits have yet to become familiar with the organization's corporate culture; they missed out on the in-person onboarding sessions, coaching, network events and training programmes.

Some organizations set up a buddy system in which new employees could approach a specific colleague with their questions. Other organizations introduced extra office days for new hires or wrote detailed introductions and manuals on work processes. In some cases, important meetings or protocols were recorded so that young employees could refer back to them if necessary. But it was still making the most of a bad situation.

GROWING IS A JOINT ENDEAVOUR

One consequence of that precarious condition is that 54 per cent of the Generation Z employees around the world are considering leaving their current company within the next 12 months, according to the recent Young Professionals survey by the training company Careerwise. Why? Because they are dissatisfied with their jobs. If they feel they are stagnating rather than growing, as an employer you are going to lose them.

Generation Z lives, works and studies in groups. Personal growth is also a group process, with input from their manager and their co-workers. A striking finding from the survey is that support in tricky situations and back-up from managers is seen as crucial. Young people are ambitious, but they also want that security. If a young employee feels they are not getting ahead, there is a bigger risk that they will hand in their resignation. That is why letting them experience that growth is at least as important as the training offered by the employer, as this survey shows.

Personal development is more important than ever for our young people in our rapidly changing world. Discovering and developing their talents, learning new skills and doing training courses are high up on their wish list. I have to agree with them.

It should be noted that this does not just apply to young employees. A survey among our clients shows that what staff missed most during the pandemic was the chance to learn and to grow. While you can do countless courses online from home, you also learn a lot from one another. A study by Maastricht University estimated that 85 per cent of what you learn at the office is picked up informally. That is forgotten sometimes. When coming up with a policy for hybrid work with a lot of working from home, you need to find alternatives for this, such as sessions in which staff share problems and solutions.

THE WORLD'S YOUR OYSTER (FOR WORK)

Andries told me enthusiastically about his latest acquisition during a Zoom session. He is 29 and works as a young economist for a venture capital fund in London. His girlfriend Hanne, who now also works in London after jobs in Madrid and Amsterdam, is finalizing a spreadsheet with price agreements. Cypress trees sway in the background and I can hear the sound of cicadas. Andries and Hanne have rented a house in the Italian countryside as a base to work for the next few months.

Andries and Hanne are not unusual. For many young professionals, the pandemic was the final push in a decision to go for a life as digital nomads. For their book *Digital nomads. In Search of Freedom, Community and Meaningful Work in the New Economy*, Rachael A. Woldoff and Robert C. Litchfield interviewed 70 location-independent millennials who had fled the cities, offices and rat race in search of more autonomy and mobility and a better quality of life. They concluded that while digital nomads don't share a physical location with colleagues, they still enjoy collaborating with people from a variety of companies, industries and countries. They derive their personal and professional satisfaction from such anytime-anywhere collaboration. Will we see an increase in the number of digital nomads? When the pandemic hit us, expats moved back home *en masse* to continue working from there. International lobby groups in London, New York and Brussels saw their members' employees leave the city for long periods.

The opportunities for young employees will increase tremendously when hybrid work becomes the norm. That elite dream job a three-hour commute from your home becomes a feasible option if you can work from home three weeks a month and stay locally in a hotel for the fourth week. Working for a start-up in Silicon Valley while based in Antwerp, or vice versa, will be serious options. Organizations can expect high rates of staff turnover now that young people no longer need to leave their desk or home to change jobs.

And finally...

Will companies start presenting themselves as "the most hybrid place to work" in the war for talent? It is certainly no longer enough to boast about being "a great place to work". You can no longer win professionals' hearts and minds with a crèche, ironing service, well-filled fridge and ping-pong table. Only organizations that take a smart approach to remote work and mental wellbeing will have a strong enough position in the labour market to attract the best young professionals in their own country and across the world.

In the next chapter, I will be taking a step back and looking at the period before we start work — I will be focusing on education. How can we make education fit better with the world of work? How can teachers spark a growth mindset in young people? But first I will consider the young people themselves and the challenges and opportunities they face.

CHAPTER 6

THE FUTURE IS ALREADY HERE

WHY BRAIN-FRIENDLY POLICIES ARE ALSO FOR THE YOUNG

Jan Hoek from Rotterdam was 15 when the Second World War started. He grew up "in an awful time". He wasn't able to enjoy the liberation from the Nazis for long either because in 1946 he was called up to fight for the Dutch in the Indonesian War of Independence. By the time he returned in October 1949, he had lost ten years of his life. In an Open Letter in the summer of 2020 that went viral, Jan Hoek called on the youth of today not to give up in the face of this crisis. "What I want to say to you young people is that we lost ten years of our youth. So try to keep your spirits up for another year. After another year, you will probably be able to enjoy your young lives to the full again. I'm 94, but I'm counting on you."

Jan Hoek was not the only one to think young people did not have it that bad during the pandemic. And he was right to a certain degree, at least if you look at the surface. I too know young people who would have been happy for the crisis to go on even longer, teenagers and students who enjoyed one another's company and the opportunity to see more of their parents who were normally out of the house so much. One acquaintance described this period as "unique family time".

However, we must not generalize from these positive experiences. For many young people, the Covid period really did have a huge adverse impact on their mental wellbeing. Imagine suddenly being forced to spend hours in front of your computer without your classmates around you. Or celebrating turning eighteen in a lockdown. Missing out on the end-of-year outing, starting at university without ever getting to see your fellow students in the flesh, having to do the internship you had so been looking forward to online... The young were deprived of more things than most people. Their longing for festivals, a revival of the Roaring Twenties and a hot vax summer was indeed quite logical as social contact is as important for youngsters' development as a healthy diet.

Another reason why we should pay particular attention to the young is that the crisis came at a point when their young brains were still developing. Our brains carry on growing and our personalities keep developing up to the age of 25. That means the disruption and the way young people and their environment responded will have long-term effects. After all, many mental health problems originate in youth.

In this chapter, I will examine the challenges that young people faced in more depth, looking at the loss they have suffered in recent months in terms of learning and living. Although we need to acknowledge that just as the current brain crisis has its roots in the pre-pandemic era, so the mental wellbeing of young people was already under pressure due to several worrying trends. However, I also want to show in this chapter how the crisis can be used to increase young people's self-awareness and empathy, and prepare them to deal flexibly with changes in the future. They too can use a crisis to grow.

Finally, I will be addressing the educators. While not everyone is equally positive about the rapid switch schools made to remote learning and digitalization, hybrid education undoubtedly offers many opportunities. Could this crisis prompt a successful reset in education? I believe it could – if the brain criterion is used as the yardstick, at any rate.

Youth in times of crisis: the challenges

LOSING OUT IN LIVING

Wrapped in cotton wool

Summer 2018, a holiday chalet on the island of Texel. I am on holiday with friends — a couple and their teenage children. It's all very sociable. But on the first morning, their teenage son appears at ten o'clock and asks me indignantly, "Why are you already clearing away breakfast?" I am surprised at his tone of voice. We had all agreed to have breakfast at nine. He hadn't turned up so I assumed he didn't want breakfast or that he would make his own arrangements later in the morning.

He had different expectations. He was clearly used to being served breakfast at the table at a time of his choosing. When he asked me whether he could have a fried egg, I realized he behaved like a consumer in his own family.

What a contrast with the previous year, on a holiday with another couple. The parents and children took it in turns to lay the table for breakfast, which seemed quite natural to me. After all, a relationship with children should be a partnership, not one-way traffic. If you only let children consume — whether in the family, at school or in society at large — you will create passive creatures lacking self-discipline and willpower. Eventually, it means they will be less likely to take over the driver's seat in their lives. That has consequences for their resilience.

The child and adolescent psychologist Peter Adriaenssens came to the same conclusion: "Our society does not make enough demands on teenagers to do something in return for society. Why don't we ask teenagers to supervise a playground or maintain a green verge? See youngsters not just as consumers but also and above all as participants in society. If you do that, you give them appreciation and responsibility."

Schools and society as a whole can play an important role in encouraging participation among youngsters but I believe the primary responsibility lies with the parents. However, parents seem increasingly to be failing to show their children leadership. That worries me. 'Authority' almost seems to be a dirty word. Many children grow up wrapped in cotton wool. In the past, if we were bullied at school our parents said it would make us stronger. These days, parents immediately go to the school head. When I take my daughters to their swimming lessons, I see children aged seven who are still being undressed and dressed by their parents. These children sit on a bench and wait patiently until their parents put their shoes on. Yet most children of seven are perfectly capable of dressing themselves. Why don't we empower them?

Make no mistake, there is nothing innocent about that pampering. Our brains — and in particular the prefrontal cortex — carry on developing until we are 25. You need the prefrontal cortex to resolve problems and reduce stress and for empathy and focus. But the prefrontal cortex needs stimulation and practice to develop properly. It grows thanks to setbacks — a row with a sibling, a lousy day, a relationship that fails, a summer overshadowed by resits.

If you constantly pamper your kids, they don't get enough opportunity to train their willpower. They never have to fight for something or make an effort. They become lazy because you take everything over from them. That has implications for their future resilience and success.

I admit that many parents have a difficult time surviving in our modern-day rat race. Many parents work hard and cannot be there for their children all the time. Is that why they try to make sure that the little time they do spend with their children goes as smoothly as possible, and prefer to avoid confrontation? Or do the beautifully lit, eternally cheerful images of parenthood that we see every day on social media mean that many parents are setting the bar unrealistically high and aiming for an unattainably picture-perfect family life?

The many opinions on parenting that they are constantly bombarded with reinforce that effect. But allow me to add one more parenting tip: parents have a responsibility to arm their children for the future. They don't do that by pampering them. They do it by inspiring their children to be heroes from a young age, to take the initiative and to assume ownership. They do it by bringing their children up with a growth mindset, by encouraging lifelong learning and by giving them the tools to make connections with others. Parents should not look to the school to do all this.

It also means that when you are with your children, you should give them your full attention because these are not tasks you do on the side. So after work, play a board game together and have real conversations rather than sitting in front of Netflix every evening.

No time for this? Take the example of my first holiday in Texel. My friends' teenage children treated me to pancakes and a fresh fruit salad. I could have a lie-in precisely because the parents had invested in their upbringing. It pays to increase children's willpower.

Unfortunately, the coronavirus crisis has made the effects of the 'cotton-wool upbringing' worse. The pandemic and associated measures have deprived youngsters of opportunities to train their willpower for a year and a half — and counting. They were no longer able to practise their hobbies, they could not socialize and screen time exploded. Some university students spent the entire first year studying remotely after they had finished secondary school without the usual end-of-year outing or prom. Missing out on such occasions also means they missed out on being caught smoking on a school trip to Rome, feeling lonely in student halls or being stood up after an exciting night at a festival. These are the experiences that train your willpower. They are the rough and tumble that give life its sparkle.

The lack of such experiences over a long period will undoubtedly have an impact on young people's wellbeing. I expect that these young people will find it harder to persevere with their studies and that they might also find it harder to resist the temptation of drugs, alcohol and other stimulants.

For that reason, I think it would have been best to vaccinate the young first in the vaccination campaign. That would have let them pick up the thread of their lives more quickly in these formative years.

Unfortunately that could not be done, of course, with the inevitable consequences. So it will be important for young people to encounter challenges again in this post-Covid era. Parents and teachers can help by encouraging them to experiment and build up more willpower. No, that doesn't mean we should send them off to large festivals or on holiday partying in countries with high infection levels; it does mean we should give our youngsters space to explore the possibilities for themselves and craft their own lives in a trial-and-error process. A community engagement crisis plan is what child psychiatrist Bie Tremmery calls it. "Remove all the 'Keep off the grass' signs and put up barbecues everywhere, for example. Such minor acts are sometimes all you need to let groups function again." Shred the cotton-wool wrapping!

LOSING OUT IN LEARNING

In addition to modern parenting styles, I am concerned about the quality and relevance of our primary and secondary schools. My gut feeling has been confirmed by international comparative studies such as PISA, TIMSS and PIRLS for some years now. The performance of pupils in the Flemish region of Belgium has been declining, and there are big differences between schools and between pupils. Too much depends on the engagement of individual teachers. Some put their all into their job whereas others are slackers who chose teaching because it offered job security.

If that is the shaky starting position for schools when they have to close and switch to remote education for weeks on end, it is hardly surprising that education experts were soon worrying about the learning loss children would incur due to the crisis. The experts based their warnings on studies of lengthy teacher strikes and the loss of learning that occurs each summer during the two-month holiday. However, it was not clear for some time whether their predictions would prove correct because for the first time in history children were being offered online education.

Now we have the data. Since the start of the pandemic, more than 70 per cent of the young people in education or combining education with work have suffered from the closure of schools, universities and training centres, according to an analysis by the International Labour Organization (ILO). Its report 'Youth & COVID-19: Impacts on jobs, education, rights and mental wellbeing' states that 65 per cent of the respondents said they had learned less since the start of the pandemic because of the switch from traditional teaching to online and remote education during the lockdown. Despite their efforts to carry on studying and take courses, half were expecting to get behind in their studies and 9 per cent thought they would fail. The situation was even worse for young people in low-income countries, who have less access to the internet, a lack of equipment and often no room to study at home.

Some young people coped better than others, and I see various reasons why. Obviously, youngsters who did not have their own laptop or a good internet connection were harder to reach. And it is a lot easier to focus on the course material if you have your own room than when the entire family is working around the kitchen table. But resilience played a role too. Young people with plenty of self-discipline and self-awareness were better at organizing their schoolwork than others of their age who were easily distracted or lacked the intrinsic motivation. And it also helped if their parents were able to assist them.

If those facilitating factors were absent, remote education was a tough call. But the education sector itself bears considerable responsibility for the failure of online teaching.

Not prepared for digitalization

"The French lesson started half an hour late again because our teacher couldn't log in." "The teacher spends the whole time talking; there's no interaction. I can't concentrate anymore and we're only halfway through the school day." I constantly heard such stories when I was out on my lunchtime walks during the pandemic and came across children from the neighbourhood.

When COVID-19 forced schools to switch to new forms of teaching with remote education and extensive use of digital technology, not all schools and teachers had the right tools and skill set to adapt to the new setup. According to an OECD study from 2018, fewer than 40 per cent of educators felt prepared for using digital technology in teaching. A survey by the Belgian youth expertise centre Ambrassade revealed that 72 per cent of the 2,400 youngsters who responded thought fewer than half their teachers were good at teaching online.

There were also huge differences between teachers. In an international study, educational innovation professor Jo Tondeur examined how teachers experienced the sudden switch to remote learning during the pandemic and what those experiences meant for the future. "Some teachers had the feeling that it all went too fast and they didn't have sufficient IT knowledge. They carried on teaching in the same way, only now in front of a camera. The result was groggy pupils after seven hours staring at a screen. But there were also teachers who embraced the new options. They discovered new tools, gave their pupils autonomy and changed their teaching style, adopting more of a coaching role. That group *was* able to make good use of the technology."

Personally, I find that very disappointing. I expect something more from a sector that is so heavily subsidized and on which the younger generation's future depends. "Education should function like a good hospital," according to education expert Martin Valcke in *Psychologies*: "With highly qualified, outstanding personnel, an innovative policy and supported by top-of-the-range technology. But what do we do? We give schools cheap computers, don't have any systematic programme for increasing professionalization, don't let teachers specialize further... If a hospital were to function like some schools, there'd be some places where you would risk people dying."

Not ready for the future

According to the World Economic Forum, 65 per cent of six-year-olds will eventually do jobs that do not yet exist. A study by the consultancy firm McKinsey estimates that the current rate of change is ten times faster than during the Industrial Revolution and the scale is 300 times bigger. The coronavirus crisis increased the realization that the world is changing fast. That is why the OECD called on countries to intensify their efforts to promote lifelong learning. "Education that is primarily geared to transferring knowledge is no longer relevant and worthwhile when the half-life of that knowledge is declining each year," writes Bieke Claes, the former CEO of Belgian American business facilitator BelCham, in an opinion piece.

As regards lifelong learning, the EU average for people aged between 25 and 64 doing a formal study is 9.2 per cent. However, there are big differences between countries. The available budgets for lifelong learning in the Netherlands are ten times higher than in Flanders. In Australia, you need to take regular accreditation tests to demonstrate your skills as an accountant or pilot are still up to date.

A lack of a tradition in lifelong learning means that many people lack the ability to learn new skills. If they see a job vacancy, they focus immediately on what they are not (yet) able to do and they don't go for the jobs where the gap between their current skill set and the required skills is too large. They 'forget' that they could also draw up a plan to grow.

Many teachers — the ones who are supposed to be teaching our young people a growth mindset — suffer from the same problem.

There is hardly any investment in their development during their career as teachers. Valcke: “We saw what consequence that had during the period of remote education: not all teachers were able to work with computers.”

Teacher training is a very different matter in Scotland, for example, where the degree is not the end point but the starting point. Teachers then have to specialize, do a probation year and get a professional update every five years. It is hardly surprising that teaching as a profession is highly regarded there.

NEEDING PSYCHOLOGICAL HELP

In addition to getting behind in their education and life experiences, young people’s mental wellbeing also suffered from the pandemic. This effect should not be underestimated. Newspapers were full of reports of teachers sounding the alarm. I remember a despondent form teacher who had had to deal with three suicide attempts in the same class.

This development too can be traced back to before the pandemic. Professor Inez Germeys of KU Leuven University has been studying the mental wellbeing of young people for some years in the SIGMAproject. Her study in 2018 of 2,000 schoolchildren aged 12, 14 and 16 showed that 66 per cent had experienced some mental health problems. A fifth of the respondents even reported moderate to severe psychological problems such as depressive feelings, problems sleeping or a death wish. The same study showed a clear association between youngsters’ mental wellbeing and their social skills. Adolescents with strong social skills who were able to practise those skills and enjoyed a lot of support from the people around them felt distinctly more at ease with themselves.

Germeys carried out another survey during the coronavirus crisis. She assumed that if social skills were so important to young people's wellbeing, the lockdowns with the restrictions on social contacts could have had a huge impact. Yet her survey in April 2020 showed no deterioration in youngsters' mental health. In fact, their feelings of anxiety had even fallen slightly on average. It seemed that a break from all the external pressure had done them some good.

I can understand that. However, a quiet period in lockdown with little stimulation is not good for the long-term development of children and young people. The young need to get out, interact with people in person and go through life experiences. Only then will they be able to grow as people, which is a prerequisite for mental wellbeing.

Indeed, young people felt much worse during the second lockdown. The lack of social contacts for such a long time started to weigh heavily. The YoungMinds charity in the UK carried out a series of surveys of the young during the pandemic. When asked during the second lockdown what the biggest problems were, the respondents mostly cited loneliness and isolation, worries about their work for school, college or university and the loss of their daily routine. Many youngsters were also concerned about the future. While some were optimistic about the roll-out of the vaccine, others were afraid that restrictions would be relaxed too soon, leading to the reintroduction of stringent measures in the future.

Specifically, 75 per cent of the respondents said they were finding the second lockdown tougher than the first, and 67 per cent thought that the pandemic would have a negative effect on their mental health in the long term. This included younger people who had experienced a death in the family or a traumatic episode during the pandemic, and youngsters who were worried about whether their friendships would recover or who were concerned about the loss of education or their employment opportunities.

It was not only the long period without social contact that was a problem: the lack of prospects and the ambiguity on what rules applied to students sharing a house, for example, did not help either. What is more, young people felt no one was listening to them. Most measures were not designed with them in mind. University students in particular had the impression they had been forgotten.

"There is genuinely nothing to look forward to at the moment. Nothing to keep you going for now because it might get better soon. After the exams, we'll go back to sitting at our computers every day. There is no breathing space, no hope, nothing to hold onto. We can't keep this up," said one student.

This is all very concerning. We already know that most psychological complaints originate when people are in their teens and twenties. The mental problems that young people are experiencing now could plague them long into their adult lives. In other words, this is not just an acute situation; we must look after this group in the medium and long term too.

As I mentioned earlier, the situation was already critical before the pandemic, with 20 per cent of young people reporting moderate to severe complaints. But now the group we need to worry about has become larger — much larger. Yet the number of available beds in psychiatric institutions has not risen in line with this increasing demand. As a society, we may well find ourselves bearing the consequences of this for many years to come. That is why we need to take action now on a brain-friendly policy for our young people.

There was very little sympathy for their circumstances from some quarters. The hype around lockdown parties and exuberant holidays served to paint young people as the main spreaders of the virus. I hope I have been able to show why we need to go easy on our youngsters: their mental wellbeing was under pressure, they suffered learning loss and they missed out on life experiences. I also think we should be more explicit in pointing out the incredible solidarity of the young during the crisis. They were the least susceptible to the virus yet they may have paid the highest price.

What about the solidarity of other generations with the young? What did we do with young people's psychological problems and cry for help? Instead of showing empathy or coming up with creative solutions, we said things like "Can't they just man up?" or "They should try harder — this isn't the war". The reactions were so extreme that when I wrote an opinion piece in support of the young, I was sent hate mail.

Why did our young people provoke such polarizing responses? It is not difficult to come up with an explanation. People often show little sympathy for mental health problems anyway, and that effect seems to be even stronger with young people. It goes against our intuitive understanding of the world to accept that young people are struggling. Shouldn't they be in the springtime of life?

Even so, it is touch-and-go whether they were the group that got the most criticism during the pandemic. It was remarkable how strict we were in our condemnation of others, even though most people applied a flexible interpretation of the rules when it suited them. But woe betide the neighbour who did the same!

In the final analysis, it should not be a competition in who suffered most, as long as we acknowledge the tough time young people had. Not that we should turn them into victims, for the crisis offers them plenty of opportunities too.

Every crisis is an opportunity, especially if you are young

"A whole generation will be lost". Plenty of experts predicted a 'lost generation'. Even the United Nations Children's Fund UNICEF spoke of this. We put this proposition to child and youth psychiatrist Peter Adriaenssens in our Better Minds at Work podcast. His answer was adamant. "It is an exaggeration and even harmful to speak of a 'lost generation'. Young people hear such language and internalize that message. Of course, some experiences have not been positive. But talking about a 'lost generation' says more about our baseline measurement and how we are now starting to find it only logical that our lives are 'perfect'."

I believe it is not only an exaggeration to speak of a 'lost generation', I would even say the opposite is true. This crisis could be a unique opportunity for our young people. Research shows that children who grow up in times of crisis are more resilient than people who only faced major challenges later on in life. Young people will inevitably have to deal with some serious things in their lives. After going through a crisis and coping with it, they will have the confidence that they will always land on their feet whatever happens. Rather than talking about a 'lost generation', we should emphasize the new challenges and ask youngsters to help us adults and collaborate with us.

In this next section, I discuss the opportunities for young people in the crisis in more depth.

"Before the coronavirus crisis, my 21-year-old son was in student accommodation, going to lectures and studying for exams in the rhythm that was imposed on him. He is not a morning person and he would complain about the morning lectures. When the education went online, he had to divide up his day and make a schedule himself. Lectures were recorded and he could view them whenever he wanted. That meant he would have a lesson marathon on Sunday afternoons sometimes, replaying some lectures at double the speed. Sometimes he got the planning wrong and I would hear him working until late in the evening. Now his schedule is in order. He has time for his partner, his university studies and his hobbies and he plays an active role in the family. He feels in control of his life. I notice that this experience has also made him more self-sufficient in other areas too. He is ready to stand on his own two feet. I was expecting him to learn that lesson when he moved out into student accommodation, but ironically it happened when he was at home in lockdown."

My colleague Hilde is proud of how her son Tijl coped with the crisis. While in previous summers she and her husband would have cracked open a bottle to celebrate her youngest son's exam results, this year they drank a toast to his resilience. The family sees a degree as important, but Hilde is even more impressed with how her son has dealt with the stress and taken control of his own life.

Hilde is not alone. Speaking to the Belgian newspaper *De Standaard,* secondary school head teacher Eddy De Schryver said: "What are we learning today at school? Well, independence, taking responsibility, the value of human relationships, solidarity with other generations, the realization that as a young person you are not alone in the world..." Isn't that great?

How was Hilde's son able to find the strength to deal with all these changes so smoothly? Hilde asked him. "I saw how Dad and you had made radical changes to your lives, how you'd got to grips with all that new technology to carry on with your work and stay in contact with friends and family, how you looked for ways to make things as pleasant as possible and never seemed to panic. If you could manage, then so could I."

It is quite clear that the way parents deal with stress and change affects how their children cope. Setbacks are a normal part of life, but sometimes we seem to have forgotten this and parents do tend to dramatize the everyday ups and downs of their children's lives. One failed exam and you can forget that glowing career, one dubious girlfriend/boyfriend and you have ruined your future. Young people copy such strategies. If parents overreact in a stressful situation, their children are likely to do the same. The fact that Hilde did not panic and coped flexibly with the changes inspired her son to do the same.

I heard about another specific technique for enhancing your children's resilience from Peter Adriaenssens. If a young person comes to him because they have broken up with their boyfriend or girlfriend and they feel depressed, he asks them to draw their family tree. They have to take that family tree to a relative and ask them one question: "Which people in the family tree have gone through hard times?" A bankruptcy for example, or a miscarriage, a serious illness or a divorce. The second question they have to ask is: "What did they do to get over it?" These stories of resilience in the family are always incredibly inspiring. They show that everyone goes through tough times but they usually pull through. What is more, previous generations could not always call on the assistance of psychotherapists. They had to draw on their inner strength.

Parents bear a major responsibility for the resilience of their children. Adriaenssens uses the metaphor of the chair. "As a parent, you want life to be kind to your child. If you say, 'Oh no! The world is going to pot. What kind of a future will you have?', you are pulling the chair away from your child just as they sit down. You can make your child more resilient instead by focusing on their talents and emphasizing how they can respond flexibly to new situations thanks to those talents. So rather than pulling the chair away at the last moment, you are giving some more chairs they can always sit on."

That is why it is a good idea to take a step back sometimes when raising children. Ask yourself whether this reflex or reaction is beneficial for your children. Is it encouraging them to take ownership when you ask them what they want to eat as if you are offering a restaurant menu? Or would it be better to work on a weekly menu together? Is it a good idea to spend the entire evening complaining about the reorganization at work? Or would it be better to stress the interesting changes ahead? Should we keep moaning about the fact that the entire family has to share the same space to work and study? Or should we all work together on turning the attic into a study room?

YES, THEY CAN TALK ABOUT EMOTIONS!

We are not good at talking about our emotions. Yet I have been hearing for a while that young people are more open about such things than previous generations. Just as the woke generation aims to end the taboo about gender identity, so they also talk openly about mental health. It is not uncommon for people to share their panic attacks or depression on social media, and candid posts about mental wellbeing can count on a very positive response. The coronavirus crisis accelerated that trend. Youth consultant Loredana Cremery stated: "Now, if someone says things are going well we find that suspicious. I always probe further. 'Are things really going that well?' Or I talk frankly about a low point I had, for instance." Rather than a 'lost generation', perhaps they will become a particularly empathic generation capable of talking honestly about their fears and insecurities and of seeking help sooner. And capable of supporting others and cheering them up.

Furthermore, this generation is more aware of what they value because of what they missed out on during the crisis. Many young people got to know themselves much better as a result. They discovered how nice it is to take life at a slower pace for a while, and learned that life does not always need to be busy or spectacular. That is enriching. This is a generation who had to grow up fast.

Here too, parents can play a supportive role, for example by openly admitting it if you are struggling, and by encouraging your children when they share their insecurities. Whoever they choose to speak to. For example, a friend told me indignantly that her son's teacher had approached her about the fact that her son was having a hard time emotionally. "Why didn't he come to me?" she said. "I'm always telling him he can talk to me about anything." I countered that she should be proud her son had asked for help and apparently knew where to find someone who had his best interests at heart. Parents need to give their children permission to speak openly, including to others.

For society at large, it is important to have sufficient lines of communication available and that the young people (or their parents or teachers) know who they can turn to. At present, many young people can't see the wood for the trees in the professional help on offer. We need to cluster these initiatives and make them more accessible. Above all, of course, we need to make sure there is enough capacity in the mental health service. That is not the case at the moment, which is why there is so much pressure on parents and teachers.

Calling all teachers – where is the reset?

The post-Covid reset has already begun in the private sector. Hybrid work is the future. But I don't see any sign of that mental reset in our primary and secondary schools. They have mainly spent the past few months hoping for code green and a return to the old normal. While I admit that remote education was not a great success — at least, not in the form it took during the pandemic — I still see plenty of opportunities in blended learning.

For example, I once sat in on a geography lesson with one of my stepchildren. It was a wonderful lesson that the teacher had clearly put a lot of effort into. It would be such a pity if that lesson was only used once. If the geography teacher were able to put that lesson online for reuse, he would free up time to devote to other skills. Why can't we build on that in the future? Why can't we have the best of both worlds? But then people say, "Children can't learn properly from home". I don't believe that. Some aspects of teaching definitely can move online.

If the traditional approach to teaching is clearly failing to deliver, why is there so much resistance to remote education? Why has education acquired a reputation for being a slow, ponderous container ship where a change of direction takes a long time to have an effect? That is not actually so surprising. Humans have an inbuilt aversion to change. You can only be flexible if you are also resilient. However, it is hard to be upbeat about reform if your resilience has become weak. Many teachers are overworked and at their wit's end, so you need to do something about that if you want to get them on board.

But there is hope. The education sector discovered in the past year that radical change is possible. Everyone discovered how resilient they could be. While in the past schools relied heavily on traditions and habit, ideas are now being discussed that were unthinkable even two years ago. They range from letting older pupils work from home one day a week to having shorter summer holidays.

I hope that remote education 2.0 will be here to stay. It has benefits as long as you go for a hybrid mix that blends classical and digital methods. All the experts agree that remote education only does not work. Schools are not just knowledge factories; they also have an important social function. And school can be a safe haven for pupils in difficult home circumstances. But there are plenty of opportunities in blended education.

And before you start panicking about having to share your office at home with your six-year-old again, some other countries have come up with a solution to this childcare problem, with learning centres where schoolchildren can study independently with the assistance of a coach.

Based on my own experience with a doctorate in psychology, expertise in resilience and first-hand knowledge of the private sector, I would like to present some key priorities for the schools of the future.

NOT JUST A COPY OF THE TRADITIONAL APPROACH

Just as back-to-back Zoom meetings are disastrous for the productivity of adult employees, back-to-back online lessons are disastrous for the concentration of young pupils. And just as working from home should not be a copy of work in the office, so remote education should not be a copy of education in the classroom. How could schools even think of organizing remote education in this way? If you look at how companies and their staff adapted in order to keep working from home doable, it seems incredible that teachers were asking children to do something that was draining their energy.

It means you need to rethink school timetables, course material and learning processes. OECD research showed that countries that invested heavily in the digital infrastructure of their schools but failed to rethink learning processes scored worse in the international PISA rankings that countries that did do this.

Make the brain criterion the primary yardstick here. Schedule lessons that require maximum focus at times when the brain is still fully alert — in the morning, in other words. Brainstorm sessions and discussions, on the other hand, can easily be held at the end of the school day.

It is also absolutely essential to incorporate sufficient recovery time in the school day. In particular, those breaks should be scheduled to suit the brain's requirements, and not because tradition dictates that you always have a break between 10:15 and 10:30. For example, after a lesson about a difficult topic, the teacher could send the class to the park to give them time to absorb what they have learned. After a test, perhaps time should be scheduled for some yoga to reduce stress levels.

DIGITAL NATIVES — FOR REAL

The crisis has forced schools to make huge progress in digitalization. Nowadays, teachers are happy working with concepts like 'break-out rooms' and 'unmuting the class'. Meanwhile, every youngster should have their own laptop and no one should have to log in on their smartphone. How many school heads have long dreamed about further digitalization but were unable to persuade the team of teachers because of the lack of a sense of urgency?

We need to build on this impulse. More guidance is needed as well, not just for teachers but also for pupils. You can't just give each schoolchild a laptop without also making them aware of the dangers of being permanently online. One of my clients gave her ten-year-old son a smartphone during the first lockdown because he missed his friends so much. A few months later he turned out to be heavily addicted to his phone and she caught him using it at night. She got rid of the smartphone but her son had severe withdrawal symptoms for a good two months. The idea that all young people are digital natives is also not correct. Of course, they know how to upload a film to TikTok or how to play and win a video game, but they don't always have the necessary digital skills for efficient remote learning. We can only truly prepare our young people for a future in a high-tech world by investing in this.

FIRST-CLASS SOLUTIONS

Digitalization could lead to a significant improvement in the quality of the education. For example, you could record lectures by a teacher who is particularly skilled in inspiring their audience or by an international expert in a particular field. You could even use a studio with first-class production values — WeZooz Academy in Belgium is a good example. That can lead to big gains in efficiency. After all, it will allow teachers to share and swap ready-made lessons, even with colleagues in other countries. Why shouldn't your university in Belgium use a lecture by an expert at Harvard?

The time that is freed up can then be used in live discussions of the material by teachers and students, on individual feedback and on psychological support. It will also help cope with the shortage of teaching staff. The number of contact hours that students have with teachers can be reduced thanks to the pre-recorded lessons. Online test platforms with automated corrections using AI can take over much of the correcting, marking and filling in reports from teachers. That makes this a financially appealing solution too.

FREEDOM IMPLIES RESPONSIBILITY

During the coronavirus crisis, education was based on trust rather than supervision. Head teachers had to place their trust in their team, who were working from home, and give them space. Parents also had to trust that the teenagers shut in their room really were studying and not playing video games. Teachers and pupils were given more freedom, but that also implied responsibility. They had to organize their own lives to perform well. I hope this development will be sustained after the pandemic, as all these elements foster ownership and resilience.

EVERY CHILD IS DIFFERENT

According to Martin Valcke, the learning gap is the main reason why a return to the old normal would be so difficult. "The differences between pupils have become too large. That has been a trend for some while. For example, researchers in Antwerp found that some three to five-year-olds barely know 800 words whereas others in the same class use 3,500 words. Even before the pandemic, teachers could only work easily with 30 per cent of the class: one third fell behind and another third had got ahead. The crisis has intensified this increasing diversity. Only a highly individualized approach will help." The schools that fail to make the necessary reforms will be left behind, predicts Valcke.

Fortunately, a shift is already underway towards alternative teaching methods that allow for differences in levels. Educative technology is a booming business internationally. Smart technology is used to tailor exercises and assignments to pupils' individual requirements based on their performance in tests. It means that each pupil can follow a customized personal learning programme. The result is much greater diversification than you could ever get with traditional books. The learning programme is created by AI, and the teacher supervises and coaches the pupils.

From a psychology perspective, this is a good idea. Each pupil is given ownership of their own learning process. That stimulates and increases their resilience. After all, it is absurd to assume that all children of a particular age should be capable of precisely the same things and therefore be given precisely the same course material. Forcing them along the same track turns them into passive consumers of education. It is a much better idea to let pupils navigate their learning environment like they would a computer game. As soon as they have acquired certain skills, they can progress to the next level. If you focus on pupils' individual requirements, each child can develop their talents to the full.

A MARIE KONDO FOR EDUCATION

Now that it has become clear that children will not be able to make up all the learning loss, the discussion has turned to what part of the curriculum is essential and what not. Which skills do we need for the future and which are clutter? "Focus on the Christmas tree, not on the decorations," says Martin Valcke.

In an interview, Belgian education expert Dirk Van Damme said, "In a crisis, you need to critically review the entire curriculum. You need to pick out the elements that are crucial for the learning process later on and concentrate on them. I am not advocating dropping certain subjects, but this exercise does need to be carried out within individual subjects."

I think we should tackle this at a much more fundamental level, quite apart from the learning loss issue. Our education system is like Descartes' "I think therefore I am". It doesn't allow for the fact that computers are much better at thinking than humans and can store far more information. Focusing instead on authentic intelligence, the kind where we humans can make a genuine difference, requires a massive turnaround. Of course the three R's and Pythagoras' theorem remain relevant but in 2021 it is more important to be able to master new technology quickly than to know your Latin. Being able to work independently is more relevant than learning a lesson off by heart.

That also means more attention to resilience and wellbeing in the attainment targets. "You need to find a balance," says Valcke. "For example, you can focus on increasing students' vocabulary in English lessons but the English language has 200,000 words. You only need 3,000 words to manage in 90 per cent of English-language situations. Once you know them, it makes more sense to invest in developing executive functions such as perseverance or impulse control rather than learning new words." I agree. You don't make up for a learning loss by learning grammar rules at a breakneck pace, but you do by nurturing a growth mindset.

Give pupils a say in deciding what learning experiences would be challenging and meaningful for them. That not only gives them a sense of responsibility and ownership, it also boosts their self-esteem. Teachers can reinforce pupils' intrinsic motivation by rewarding effort and emphasizing areas that they are naturally interested in.

That is precisely why Better Minds at Work supports the summer schools that Bieke Claes organizes for disadvantaged children. No extra French or Maths lessons here. Instead the children get inspiring workshops on entrepreneurism and resilience, and on ownership and empathy. These are the skills we will need more than ever in the future, says Claes. “When we see that automation and robots are already taking over from humans, the loss of jobs for graduates is likely to gather pace enormously in the decades to come. The role played by our children will change to being the people steering all that capacity. The essential skills will be asking the right questions, dealing with conflicting interests and scarce resources, clearly formulating the desired objective, having a vision and, above all, being able to deploy that capacity with integrity and awareness. In other words, leadership.”

AN OPEN DOOR EVERY DAY

In the past year, the dividing line between school and free time became blurred. Parents helped out with school tasks and teachers got a unique insight into their pupils’ home circumstances.

Many parents found out about their children’s approach to learning for the first time during the pandemic. Some soon decided to take action — the private tutoring centres experienced a boom — while other parents discovered the course material was too easy for their offspring. For example, Karen prepared her daughters to skip a year at school while they were studying from home. Often in the past such discussions only take place after parents get the school report, but now parents were taking preventive measures.

Equally, remote education introduced teachers to their pupils’ private circumstances and they were better able to judge whether the children had problems at home. Parents in turn were more likely to be addressed as partners. After all, the success of remote education depended to a large extent on the cooperation of the parents. The closer relationship between teachers and parents is one of the key opportunities to come out of the coronavirus crisis.

Working from home was also an opportunity in that sense.

Children could see what their parents' jobs involved. I told my daughters that I was about to give a talk that would hopefully make people happier and now they regularly ask me at the end of my working day whether I had made people happier. They have a much better idea of what I spend my days doing. Working from home gave them a more realistic impression than coming to the office for the annual corporate family day. For teenagers in particular, this can help them when they have to make their own decisions about their degree subject and future career.

LIFELONG CURIOSITY

The blurring boundary between school and free time offers other opportunities too. Just as the sharp distinction between work and private life has become outmoded, so we need to do the same for the distinction between school time and free time. If school is where you learn and home is where you relax, children will never develop the habit of learning outside school hours. If you also offer hobbies at school, as they do in the United States, schools will get a broader, more comprehensive picture of their pupils and schoolchildren will see school as a fun environment. That will encourage them to remain curious and eager to learn even when they are not in school.

I try to encourage that inquiring mind at home in my children too. My daughters recently came home from a weekend with their father. I asked them what they had done at the weekend and they chattered away with all their news. When they had finished, the conversation stopped. So I asked them, "Aren't you curious about what Mummy did? I had a weekend too." Since then, they always ask how my weekend was. They realize that there is someone behind the Mummy facade they see. Their inquiring mind has been activated, and they will benefit from this their entire lives.

"Academic qualifications are important but they no longer guarantee you access to the labour market," says Peter Adriaenssens in the Better Minds at Work podcast. Flexibility, a growth mindset and being able to adapt to the unexpected are more important than ever in a world that is in constant flux.

This constitutes an opportunity for young people. They experienced the importance of agility and lifelong learning first hand during the pandemic. That is not just a challenge, it also has positive aspects. In the past, your academic qualifications were a limiting factor throughout your life. "Now they can reinvent themselves whenever they want," adds Adriaenssens.

Personally, I am an advocate of 'resilience vouchers' in education that you use to discuss ideas about the next ten years with a professional. Many young people never think that far ahead, but such an exercise can be very stimulating. Of course you should not start this discussion with the question 'Where do you want to be in ten years' time?' That never produces an honest answer. But you can get a lot of clarity by asking the youngster about their talents and what pastimes they are passionate about.

OPPORTUNITIES FOR ALL

Digital education can be hugely emancipatory. Research shows that children in different social groups get a different upbringing. Books often play an important role in families where the parents went to university and are affluent. There may well be a library in the home. Children in socially vulnerable families are relatively more exposed to audio-visual content on the television or their smartphone. The result is a gap in socialization and cultural baggage.

Education that is primarily based on textual sources is a shoo-in for middle-class children, but more like an away match for children from lower-income families, who first have to adapt to the way they are being taught before they can get to grips with the content.

If digital resources are used properly, such blended education offers big opportunities for young people from disadvantaged groups. The language gap can also be bridged. Professor Agirdag developed a module for social studies in seven languages. The fact that the students could study the course material in several different languages improved their performance.

The online modules offered by universities — the MOOCs mentioned earlier — also reach people who would not have this opportunity otherwise. Examples are people who want to combine study with work or care for the family, or who live in another country.

And finally...

Aged just 13, skateboarder Sky Brown was the youngest British athlete at the Olympic Games in Tokyo. Yet for a long while it was not certain that she would be able to take part. A year earlier, she had made a mistake on a large skate ramp during training and ended up in hospital, unconscious and with a fractured skull. Her parents begged her to stop skateboarding and forbade her to watch the video of her accident. But "I was fine with it," said Brown in an interview. "It's good to fall sometimes, which is why I put the clip out there on social media. My parents didn't want me to post it but I was like 'please cos it was cool'."

This is a 13-year-old who thinks a mistake is cool and who is not afraid to get back on her skateboard after an accident. Needless to say, I wiped away a tear when Brown won the bronze in Tokyo in August 2021. No way is this a 'lost' generation.

EPILOGUE

TOGETHER IN THE GREAT GLASS ELEVATOR

28 September 2021. It is precisely eighteen months since I first saw that video clip of Sarah Defrise Nirenburg. Today I make a point of replaying it. I am curious to see what effect the video has on me now... and to catch a glimpse of the Elke of one and a half years ago. Like Proust's madeleine, the film takes me back in time, to the start of the pandemic when I thought COVID-19 would be a brief, albeit far-reaching, intermezzo in my life, when I called my company's first crisis meeting, when my divorce was still ongoing and there was no new relationship on the horizon. I can only think "What a mental reset it has been" as I listen to *These are the days* by Van Morrison with the volume at the maximum. My life has changed dramatically on various fronts in the past eighteen months. For the umpteenth time.

What makes this reset particularly potent is that I did it together with so many other people — from friends to company directors, from my children's teachers to policymakers. Every day, I hear of someone for whom COVID-19 was the catalyst for a major change. People who had been on automatic pilot for years suddenly had the courage to start a new life with a new relationship, a new job and sometimes even a new country. Instead of drifting along on autopilot, they are proactively in the driver's seat of their lives and taking nothing for granted. They decide in which areas of their lives they want to move up a gear and where they prefer to put a brake on.

They tell me they have got a taste for this new approach. But — they whisper — it was the pandemic that showed them the way. The pandemic was their reset button. "What about the future?" they ask me. "Do we have to wait for another catalyst to repeat the reset?"

Of course not. I hope that *The Mental Reset* has shown you how you can reset your life without a global crisis and why that is necessary. And how you can get your family, friends, co-workers, neighbours and so on involved in this process.

If you want to carry out another reset, I recommend getting into the Great Glass Elevator — a lift that lets you observe everything clearly from a distance. In the lift you will find a reset button. Try pressing it and see what happens. First the lift will take you to the top floor with the observation deck offering panoramic views. Take a good look around on all sides. Perhaps you should bring some binoculars, spend a while there and speak to others on the observation deck. Peer down at the ground first, to see what your life, company, school or country looks like from a distance. Note what goes wrong. Do you and your partner live separate lives, are you not getting enough satisfaction out of your free time, are your employees lacking motivation, is there a fundamental problem higher up the ranks...? Determine what area you want to make changes in.

Stay on the observation deck until it gets dark and the stars come out. They represent your dreams for the future. You may not see them clearly at first. Perhaps you have to wait until the clouds have gone. But after a while, the stars will flicker with hints of what your new future could look like. More quality time with your partner, a reorganization for your company, a move to a different city... Some stars will shine brighter than others and catch your attention. Perhaps you could join them up to create your own personal constellation?

When morning arrives, step back into the Great Glass Elevator and press the reset button again. As the lift descends, check your brand-new dream for the future against the brain-friendly criterion. Do that check on four floors:

→ Does my dream give me positive energy?
→ Does this dream address my 'why'?
→ Are there enough opportunities for growth in this dream?
→ Does this dream give me room to focus on my priorities?

If the answer to any one of these questions is 'no', you take the lift back up to the top and adjust your dream accordingly. Make sure you don't shrink your dream: your revised dream should be even bigger, wilder and more ambitious.

You can only take the lift down to the basement once you can answer 'yes' to each check. This is where you make your dream something tangible. You are going to mould it as if it were a statue, a Rodin, with an eye for detail. You can use the tools in Chapter 3 for this. Once your dream is finished, carry it under your arm and walk up to the ground floor. You no longer need the lift as the dream gives you so much energy that you can easily transport your creation up the stairs. You are virtually skipping.

Once you are on the ground floor, make your dream come true. Naturally there will be sceptics, but you stayed so true to yourself in the Great Glass Elevator that your plan will virtually implement itself. Of course you may find your sculpture incurs damage. No need to worry. If that happens, the lift will be available for you to repair your creation, remould it where necessary and perhaps even embellish it. You do that in the basement, but only after you have taken another trip to the observation deck. Sometimes you will need another minor reset, or even a major reset — but make sure you always stop at those four floors on the way down.

See the clip about the Great Glass Elevator
on the Mental Reset video channel.

I hope the crisis has brought us new insights. I hope we will be able to reflect on it as individuals, families and organizations and draw on the experience to proactively make choices and take ownership of our lives. What has it taught you, how would you like things to change from now on and what do you need to do to achieve that? You could for example start discussions with your manager about hybrid work, look at how to spend more time with your family and search for ways of incorporating some 'me time' in your weekly schedule. These are minor changes that can have a major impact.

I also hope this book has shown you that taking ownership of your life is not just about the decisions you take today; it is a lifelong project. A reset is not a one-off event but something you do repeatedly. Hybrid work, for example, is not a question of drawing up a new plan for working independently of time and place, and then you're done. On the contrary, it means constantly adjusting that plan throughout your life because you will grow as a professional, your company will evolve and society will change dramatically. Flexibility is the key to success. That means acknowledging that you personally will probably not spend your entire life working for the same organization. What is more, what your job involves will probably look very different in the future. Perhaps your current job will not even exist. That is not a problem because we humans have a very special superpower: we can diversify and develop new skills. That is why I fervently hope lifelong learning will finally become the norm. Rather than getting a degree in our twenties and being saddled with that choice for the rest of our lives, we should have the courage to reinvent ourselves time and again — and be enabled to do so. This will help us leap ahead, as individuals, as companies and as society as a whole. Let the cover image encourage you to embrace change and to do so full of confidence and with an open, authentic attitude.

I wish you many fantastic mental resets!

Elke Geraerts

Relevant literature

CHAPTER 1. MAKE IT COUNT

Elke Geraerts (2017), *Better Minds: How Insourcing Strenghts Resilience and Empowers Your Brain*. Tielt: Lannoo.

CHAPTER 2. IT DEPENDS HOW YOU LOOK AT IT

Yuval Noah Harari (2017), *Homo Deus: A Brief History of Tomorrow*. New York: HarperCollins.
Yuval Noah Harari (2021), 'Lessons from a Year of Covid', *Financial Times,* available online at: https://www.ft.com/content/f1b30f2c-84aa-4595-84f2-7816796d6841
Frank Martela, Nelli Hankonen, Richard M. Ryan, & Maarten Vansteenkiste (2021), 'Motivating voluntary compliance to behavioural restrictions: Self-determination theory based checklist of principles for COVID-19 and other emergency communications', in *European Review of Social Psychology*. Advance online publication: https://doi.org/10.1080/10463283.2020.1857082
Rutger Bregman (2021), *Humankind: A Hopeful History*. London: Bloomsbury.
Jan Romein (1935), *'De dialectiek van de vooruitgang',* in: *Forum,* 4.

CHAPTER 3. BUILD BACK BETTER

Elke Geraerts (2016), *Het Nieuwe Mentaal. Hoe lef je op weg zet naar geluk en succes.* Tielt: Lannoo.
Erik Franck, 'Slaaptraining bij chronische insomnia: toepassing van het slaap-waakregulatiemodel van Borbély', in *Huisarts Nu*, 49, pp. 17-21.
Yuval Noah Harari (2019), *21 Lessons for the 21st Century*. London: Vintage.
Nassim Nicholas Taleb (2010), *The Black Swan: The Impact of the Highly Improbable.* London: Penguin Group.
Simon Sinek (2019), *Start With Why. How Great Leaders Inspire Everyone to Take Action*. New York: Penguin Group.
Glennon Doyle (2020), *Untamed: Stop Pleasing, Start Living.* London: Vermilion.
Berthold Gunster (2010), *Ja maar... Omdenken*. Lev.: Amsterdam.
Kristin Neff (2014), *Self-Compassion. Stop Beating Yourself Up and Leave Insecurity Behind.* New York: William Morrow.
Martin Seligman (2011), *Flourish. A Visionary New Understanding of Happiness and Well-being.* New York: Atria Books.

CHAPTER 4. THE BRAIN IS KEY IN THE NEW WAY OF WORKING

Microsoft (2021), 'The Next Great Disruption Is Hybrid Work – Are We Ready?', available online at https://ms-worklab.azureedge.net/files/reports/hybridWork/pdf/2021_Microsoft_WTI_Report_March.pdf
Josh Bersin (2021), 'The Joys of Hybrid

Work. Ten Things We Have Learned', available online at https://joshbersin.com/2021/05/hybridwork/
Erica Dhawan (2021), *Digital Body Language. How to Build Trust and Connection, No Matter the Distance*. New York: St. Martin's Press.
Florence Pérès (2017), *Digital detox. Minder technostress en meer focus dankzij de Touchpoints-methode*. Tielt: Lannoo.
Jitske Kramer (2020), *Werk heeft het gebouw verlaten. Anders samenwerken na de corona cultuurshock*. Amsterdam: Boom.
Carol Dweck (2007), *Mindset. The New Psychology of Success*. New York: Ballantine Books.
Lynda Gratton (2017), 'Who's building the infrastructure for lifelong learning?', available online at https://sloanreview.mit.edu/article/whos-building-the-infrastructure-for-lifelong-learning

CHAPTER 5. THE MOST HYBRID EMPLOYER OF THE YEAR

Josh Bersin (2021), 'The secret to wellbeing at work is… leadership', available online at https://joshbersin.com/2021/04/the-secret-to-wellbeing-at-work-is-leadership/#:~:text=Leadership%20is%20key%20to%20well,impact%20on%20the%20entire%20organization
Amy C. Edmondson (2019), *The Fearless Organization. Creating Psychological Safety in the Workplace for Learning, Innovation, and Growth.* Hoboken, NJ: Wiley.
Lynda Gratton (2021), 'How to do hybrid right', in: *Harvard Business Review*, available online at https://hbr.org/2021/05/how-to-do-hybrid-right
Microsoft (2021), 'The Next Great Disruption Is Hybrid Work – Are We Ready?', available online at https://ms-worklab.azureedge.net/files/reports/hybridWork/pdf/2021_Microsoft_WTI_Report_March.pdf
Rachael A. Woldoff and Robert C. Litchfield (2021), *Digital Nomads: In Search of Freedom, Community and Meaningful Work in the New Economy.* Oxford: Oxford University Press.

CHAPTER 6. THE FUTURE IS ALREADY HERE

Peter Adriaenssens (2018), *Verbolgen verbonden. Opgroeien in een complexe wereld.* Tielt: Lannoo.

WWW.LANNOO.COM

ENGLISH TRANSLATION: Clare Wilkinson, Tessera Translations BV

COVER DESIGN: Buro Blikgoed

LAYOUT DESIGN: Armée de Verre

LAYOUT: Asterisk*, Amsterdam

PHOTOGRAPH OF THE AUTHOR: Tjorven Photography

D/2022/45/134 – NUR 770 – ISBN 978 94 014 8336 0